MW00586927

Parkinson's

Life Lessons Five Years into the Journey

GERRY HILL

Copyright © 2021 Gerry Hill
All rights reserved
First Edition

Fulton Books, Inc.
Meadville, PA

Published by Fulton Books 2021

ISBN 978-1-63710-808-6 (paperback)
ISBN 978-1-63710-809-3 (digital)

Printed in the United States of America

FOREWORD

In October of 2016, I received life-changing news. I had been diagnosed with early onset Parkinson's disease at age forty-eight. In the past five years, I feel as if I have been on a unique journey. This journey has had many pitfalls and challenges, but it has also contained memorable experiences through which I have learned how to better handle my circumstances as a Parkinson's patient and work to maintain a high quality of life. I have also learned to appreciate those around me more than I have in years past. My family has been an amazing source of support through these first five years of my diagnosis, and I am blessed to work in a school containing some of the most caring and compassionate faculty and staff members anywhere.

In October 2020, I began to get the idea to write this book. I wanted it to be a record of my journey and a detailed account of my diagnosis. Since starting this book back then, it has evolved into something else. I have found the writing to be quite therapeutic for me. It has helped me come to grips with my own failures and missteps along the way in these past few years. As I finish with this project, I know my journey with Parkinson's will continue. It is my sincere hope that I have learned something through these writings that will keep me centered and on track for a successful life in the years to come. I also hope that others who either have Parkinson's or support someone who does can take some encouragement from my experiences and apply some of the lessons I have learned to their own lives. If my story helps at least one other person have a more comfortable and productive journey, then I will consider this project a rousing success. Even if that does not happen, I can still appreciate what I have learned and work to make the next five years even better than my first five!

PART 1
The Backstory

CHAPTER 1

Golf Can Be a Real Pain

"You have early onset Parkinson's."

Stunned silence and disbelief followed those words from Dr. Dinesh Raju, a neurologist at the Gwinnett Clinic in Lawrenceville, Georgia. Did I really just hear that? There must be some kind of mistake. I'm only forty-eight years old! Parkinson's is what seventy- and eighty-year-olds get. Not me!

"I'll give you some time to talk things over with your wife, and then we'll discuss what things will be like going forward."

With those simple words, Dr. Raju stepped out into the hallway, closing the door behind him but ushering a new life scenario into my existence. "Going forward," he said? I guess that is better than going backward!

I still could not believe what I had just heard. The tears found their way out as my newly revealed neurologically challenged brain was spinning in the small medical room. How could this be? What have I done wrong? All these questions would be dealt with over time, but at the moment, they seemed almost as unsolvable as a million-piece jigsaw puzzle of a picture of the calm Atlantic Ocean—with maybe a few hundred pieces missing. I guess I had to start somewhere, so in my best "find the edge pieces first" mentality, I started thinking about how this all started and how I had come to this stunning revelation in a small medical exam room in Georgia. I hoped that by looking back, this would all make a bit more sense. In the end, it probably did help to look back and see the journey that

I had traveled as well as the new and more challenging journey that was ahead of me.

*****

Decisions, decisions. Hit the driver? Be safe with a 3-wood? Challenge the water hazard? Normally, an established golfer would engage in these very mental gymnastics as they stand on the first tee box ready for competition. Let's be perfectly clear…these are not an issue for me on the golf course as I can only dream of calling myself an "established golfer." My decisions are more along the lines of, "Do I want to shank this drive into the woods on the right or duck hook this one into the tall weeds on the left?" While these are different decisions, they must still be made while on the opening tee box of the 2016 Blackberry Cobbler Open at Apple Valley Golf Club in Lake Lure, North Carolina, on a beautiful June day.

I guess a little context would be appropriate at this point, lest you begin to think you have started reading the wrong book. My Parkinson's adventure began on the first tee box of an annual golf outing contested between Cliff Shelton, Tim Vick, Jerry Spiceland, and me—the Blackberry Cobbler Open. This nonprofessional (understatement of the year) golf event featured teams of Mr. Spiceland and me taking on Coach Shelton and Coach Vick in a three-day golf extravaganza in which the stakes were critical—the losing team had to buy the winning team servings of the world's best blackberry cobbler and ice cream at a local restaurant on the banks of a beautiful river flowing through the laid-back downtown portion of Lake Lure.

After struggling through the opening thirty-six holes on day 1, Team Hill-Spiceland trailed by a fairly massive fifteen points (using a modified scoring system awarding different levels of points for varying scores on a hole), but we were determined to make a dramatic comeback on day 2 as we headed over from the Rumbling Bald Resort course to the Apple Valley course. Today, we had decided, would be different. Of course, "different" could mean something as simple as "making contact with the golf ball in such a way as to be able to locate it without an organized search party."

"How about a little inspiration off the first tee?" Mr. Spiceland joked, channeling his inner Jack Nicklaus.

"Age before beauty!"

And with that, we were underway, after a "brief" search for a golf ball (or two) in the rough along the right-hand side of the opening fairway. The round was progressing nicely as Team Hill-Spiceland began to slowly chip away at the Team Shelton-Vick lead through the opening nine holes. We headed to the back nine with a sense of growing confidence, praying that this was not just false bravado but, instead, an actual comeback. Then it came, the moment of truth, a dynamic moment that rings clearly in my mind even all these years later.

After a decent drive (defined as one that was over two hundred yards and findable rather quickly), I was faced with a fairly simple layup shot on this long par-5 tenth hole. Grabbing my 3-wood, I aimed for a clear spot down the left side of the fairway, hoping to just have a wedge into a rather large green. In my state of delirium from having hit the fairway for once, did I dare even consider the possibility of making a legitimate birdie or, worst-case scenario, a par?

At the moment of contact, instead of experiencing the expected joy of striking a golf ball cleanly and crisply and on line, a twinge of pain gripped my left shoulder, causing an immediate release of the club as it went sailing a few yards to the left, much to the delight and entertainment of my playing opponents. As I recall, this was the first time I had cursed in front of colleagues. Instead of changing the mood, I think the "choice words" caused both Coach Shelton and Coach Vick to double over with laughter, at least at first.

"That might be the farthest your 3-wood has ever gone!" chirped Coach Shelton.

"You got *all* of that one!" chimed in Coach Vick.

Even I brushed it off with as much of a "calm, cool, and collected" veneer as I could muster and even got a bit of a laugh out of it as the initial shock of the pain subsided some over the next few minutes. While trying to get through the experience, my golf game suffered a bit. There would be no miraculous tenth-hole birdie or even a par, as the shanked 3-wood did not serve me well. I considered myself lucky to have gotten a double bogey 7 on that turning point of a hole.

Considering the circumstances, the rest of the back nine was fairly tolerable. After starting the day with such a deficit, my team had made some progress. Instead of being fifteen points behind, we were "only" nine points behind after the first eighteen holes of the day. Round 2 and the continuation of our planned staggering comeback were still to come. My body, though, had other plans in mind.

Upon arriving back at our condo after a grueling thirty-six-hole day, we all crashed and got ready for dinner. Steaks would soon be on the grill, and the world's largest baked potatoes were soon ready for consumption. The "grilling," though, was not just limited to the steak preparation. Coaches Vick and Shelton made sure to "remind" Mr. Spiceland and me about the scores on the course for the day and the "commanding" twelve-point lead they had going into the final day of competition—thirty-six holes to decide the championship of the open. Trying to be a good sport about it all (especially after the "colorful" tenth-hole commentary I provided), I took the jabs in stride but began paying more attention to the jabs I was experiencing in my shoulder. The pain was coming back, and my left arm seemed a bit "jittery." That was the word I used that night while talking to my wife on the phone. We were both convinced that it was not really a big deal and that it was just a strain or something. Looking back at those moments with around four or five years of advanced perspective, I can see more clearly now that this was probably the first manifestation of something that was about to come into my life and change my perspective on a lot more things than just my golf game and an occasional shoulder pain.

It was decided that I would simply try to take it easy on the final day of the trip and not make things any worse. As I saw it, at least I now had a built-in excuse for the failed state of my golf game. While the validity of that "excuse" was challenged by my opponents in the pen, at least I would know going in that if I played badly (a likely scenario considering my overwhelming lack of talent, even in a fully healthy state), I could blame my inadequacies on some external factor beyond my control. Of course, had I gone out the next morning and fired a career-best round in the first eighteen holes of the day, then what would I say? Maybe I should injure myself more often? Needless to say, I was spared from solving that predicament.

While the prize for the champions of the outing was delicious blackberry cobbler (made even more delicious, according to Coach Shelton, by the fact that I paid for his enormous serving), the final rounds on the course brought me a heaping helping of humble pie as our deficit grew throughout the day. Twelve points became seventeen…then twenty…then… Well, I stopped counting when I ran out of fingers and toes. My shoulder did not react well to the two rounds of golf, and I was convinced that the likelihood of some kind of injury was increasing. I even tried to use a "sore shoulder" as an excuse to not pick up the check for the cobbler, but that didn't work at all. Now besides my golf game being put on hiatus for a bit, I had to face the always fun prospect of going to the doctor to see how bad this really was. If only the first diagnosis had been correct!

CHAPTER 2

What Are You Afraid Of?

It has been said, famously, that the only thing we have to fear is fear itself. I would like to add some new items to that list: taking your car to the mechanic and hoping they don't find a whole gamut of items to fix, filing your taxes when buried under a swath of W-2 forms in a crazy year like 2020, and attending a gender reveal event. Well, okay, that last one's probably not in the same ballpark as the others, but you get the picture. Some events naturally bring with them more trepidation than others and are the source for great stress in the lives of many. This is how it is for me when going to the doctor without really knowing what's wrong. Sure, if you have a cold or the flu or you've broken a bone, you know what to expect when you see a physician, but to walk into a doctor's office and only be armed with vague statements such as "I just haven't felt like myself lately" or "Things have just been weird lately, and everything seems a bit off" brings about a feeling of uncertainty for some like me.

Naturally, then, when I entered my family doctor's office to have someone check me out, I was a bit concerned. In the back of my mind, I was "pretty sure" that I had a pinched nerve or, in the worst-case scenario, a damaged rotator cuff. After a brief exam and some stretching and twisting of muscles that brought about some facial expressions only an impressionist painter could appreciate, I was a bit relieved to hear an initial diagnosis that seemed to agree with my own "expert" diagnosis. Dr. Whiteneck was "pretty certain" (a medical term that I'm sure gets overused every day across the country) that I had strained a muscle in my shoulder and that there was a potential for some rotator cuff impairment. He recommended a chiropractic visit to determine the extent of any damage and gave me a referral for a number of physical therapy sessions to work out the area of my left shoulder in order to strengthen it back to its original state. I left the office with a bit of a sigh of relief, but I wasn't exactly looking forward to getting bent into the shape of a pretzel at the chiropractor's office.

A couple of days later, it was time for the "manipulation" (a chiropractic term that I think loosely means "to be folded and bent like a piece of origami art") at Dr. Randy's office near my home in Braselton. At least going into this visit, I knew the source of the problem and had a decent idea of what the treatment was going to entail. That settled my nerves—a bit!

Within ten minutes of filling out the forms that I think had me sign away all my legal rights to everything and promising not to scream bloody murder or physically strike the doctor at any point during the visit, I was on the table and ready to begin. After only a few minutes of observation and having my face planted in the traditional chiropractor's table opening that stares directly at the floor, the words that I knew were coming were uttered.

"Just relax!"

Oh, sure! Relax! That'll be easy! It's the same as being told not to think about purple elephants, and of course, that's all that comes to mind at the moment. By the time I could get the full picture of the odd-colored pachyderm developed in my head, the first adjustment was made. In a bizarre sensation of initial discomfort followed by an overwhelming sense of relief and bliss, I went from almost uttering the same words from the tenth hole with my 3-wood in hand to a strangely curious feeling of being by a babbling brook on a cool autumn day.

"You okay?" came the voice of Dr. Randy, interrupting my momentary solace by the soothing waters.

"I think so" was the only response I could come up with at the time, but it seemed the right thing to say in the moment.

The next few minutes had me go through a couple of more adjustments that brought a bit more relief to the situation and then a short five-minute "rest" on a rolling massage table that I now want to have in my living room on a permanent basis. Things seemed to be headed in the right direction after this initial late June visit. The plan was in place. I would come back to be mangled (or was that "manip-ulated"?) a couple more times over the next two to three weeks, and then I would start some physical therapy sessions in mid to late July that would last for about five to six weeks. That original plan, while longer than I had originally hoped for, seemed manageable and, at least, had a definite end point to it.

There would be no golfing, no cursing at 3-woods, no hour-long searches for golf balls in the woods during this "downtime" and rehab. I would miss the open fairways (notice how that was appropri-ately worded?), the wide-open spaces, the thirty-foot putts for triple bogey, and even having to pick up the check for an occasional treat of blackberry cobbler for opponents who took way too much delight in reminding me of how badly they beat my team on the course that weekend. Instead, I now knew that I could (or should) place my focus on the more daunting task of preparing for my doctoral pro-gram comprehensive exam coming up in August. All my coursework was done, and it was time to face the next step in the process—a step that would take me from simply being a doctoral student to becoming an official dissertation candidate. Now that I think about it, maybe this would be a good time to add another item to my list of things to fear!

CHAPTER 3

Tests and Other Examinations

There are all kinds of clubs one can join. Health clubs are especially popular in January of each year as thousands of people declare that *this* is the year they will shed those unwanted pounds or get in shape to run a 5K race. Book clubs offer anyone who chooses to participate an opportunity to be more well-read on popular literature of the time (or at least be able to tell their friends that they are currently reading the same book as Oprah Winfrey or some other celebrity). Jelly of the Month clubs are for those so inclined to have wonderful spreads and delicacies delivered right to their doorstep every thirty days for some "reasonable" price. Of course, we can't forget country clubs! Where would all our world's business dealings take place if we didn't have open layouts of eighteen holes of golf where executives can glad-hand their constituents and bask in the glory of making an 8 on a par-3 hole at the same time?

I've been a member of a couple of health clubs and received some benefits from them. Even though I teach English for a living, I've never really had the desire to be a part of a book club. Maybe it's that I don't like the idea of some celebrity suggesting my reading list. I won't even talk about the Jelly of the Month club! I don't want to end up having a Clark Griswold meltdown on Christmas Eve. Of course, making a teacher's salary prevents me from joining some prestigious country club. Come to think of it, though, it's probably best that my "amazing" golf talents are not on display in a location where a trademarked shank of a 3-wood could find its way into the window of a ten-million-dollar home, leaving me with an incredible bill to pay as well as massive embarrassment.

However, there is one "club" that I somehow knew I would eventually join. It's a club that, once I was admitted, nobody else on this planet could ever become a member of. This club has roots all the way back into the 1940s and 1950s. This "club" is the "doctoral club" formed exclusively by the male members of the Donald L. Hill family. My older brother, John, was the first to join the club after my dad established it many years ago with his PhD from Vanderbilt. My younger brother, Stephen, joined the club next as he finished his doctorate at the University of Alabama. Now it was my turn to join and be able to say, in my best Darth Vader voice, "The circle is now complete" as I pursued my EdD in curriculum and instruction at Piedmont College.

Starting in 2015, I was admitted into the Piedmont College doctoral program and spent the next eighteen months working through the coursework required to get the stage of the comprehensive exam, or comps. While the time commitment was pretty extensive for the program and I think I read more books in those eighteen months than I had ever read in my life up to that point, the classes were not as bad as I had originally thought they would be, and I moved through the progression with very few issues. Before long, I had made it through the final class period and was headed toward a three-week prep time to get ready for the comprehensive exam. This exam was a "survive and advance" type of test that one had to pass in order to start the dissertation process. For me, my comps day was set for the middle of August in 2016, about six weeks after my crushing defeat in the Blackberry Cobbler Open. I figured maybe the Lord was trying to tell me that I had spent too much time on the golf course and not enough time studying, so he "arranged" for my shoulder issue to come forward so that I'd be forced to stay home and study. That was just what I did, but book knowledge wasn't the only thing I learned in the process.

*****

Having left Dr. Randy's chiropractic office with a card showing the date of my first physical therapy session in just a few days, I called the rehab facility to see what I could expect. Their description of the visits did not sound too imposing. In a way, I was actually kind of looking forward to the visit so that I could get one step closer to getting my shoulder fixed and having things back to some semblance of normalcy. Little did I know that what was lying ahead in just a matter of a short few weeks would alter my definition of "normal" forever.

I pulled into the parking lot of the rehab facility with a strong sense of confidence. This was going to go well, the treatment was going to be a success, and life would soon be good once again. Not so fast! I was greeted by a very pleasant nurse who helped me through all the paperwork and even gave me a tour of the facility, showing me all the "devices of torture" (her words, not mine) that they used for various treatments. She then took me to the treatment room and explained that the first step in my treatment was going to involve electronic stimulation of the area on and around my shoulder. That didn't sound too bad. I've seen professional athletes getting stimulation treatments, and they did not seem to be a big deal. Obviously, I had never been hooked up to one of these devices before.

In just a matter of minutes, I had what looked like an oversize heating pad strapped to my shoulder, upper arm, and upper-left portion of my back. This same pleasant nurse then proceeded to tell me that I would feel a "bit of a tingle" once she turned on the device. She said the entire process would take about eight to ten minutes and that the degree of intensity of the "tingle" would vary from "almost undetectable" to "quite significant." I'm not sure I ever endured the "almost undetectable" stage, but I am quite sure I experienced the "quite significant" stage of the proceedings. Imagine a nest of angry red wasps landing on your left shoulder and stinging you while you are strapped helplessly to a chair, watching the entire process. At least the "wasp attack" only lasted for a few seconds at a time, and soon the entire ordeal was over. Time to move on to the next "stage."

After removing the pad from my shoulder, the nurse took me over to a machine designed to test my flexibility, and we soon discovered that, injury or not, I did not have very much. It was a challenge to move my arm and shoulder through a simple progression of exercises. At the time, I did not think much of the problems as it was still my first visit and the first time I had tried to work such a machine. Surely, it would get easier. In hindsight, this should have been more of a red flag for me. Something was not right.

I concluded my first visit by going over to an item called a finger wall. The device was about the length of a yardstick and was mounted on the wall so that the lower end was about waist-high off the floor and stretched upward. On this device were several ridges about an inch or so apart. The nurse called them rungs. My job was to place my left hand at the bottom of the device and then walk my fingers up the rungs as far as possible before running out of mobility. Sounds simple enough. Then I tried it. Not so simple. I managed to get about a third of the way up the rungs before experiencing a "stuck" sensation. "No problem," the nurse said. "Just try again."

I repeated the process until I had done ten reps on the finger wall. Each time, my threshold was about the same point. I could only get a third of the way up the wall. The nurse said that I had done well, but I wasn't so sure. She reminded me, though, that nobody's first visit is ever entirely successful. It takes time to get through the process and repair the damage done in my shoulder. Deep down inside, I knew what she was saying was true. That didn't mean that I had to like it or accept it. My life was too busy to spend any more time than absolutely necessary to get better. Let's just say that wasn't the last time that I was told time would be important to me.

*****

July soon turned to August 2016, and the date for doctoral comps was closing in. One of my cohort buddies and I got together one afternoon for a study session. What was supposed to be about a one-hour session turned into a four-hour marathon, but we learned more than we could probably ever use or need to know on the exam. At least, I'm sure I can say I learned something, but it wasn't just a list of terms or names of educational philosophers and their respective theories. I learned that something new was happening, and I wasn't 100 percent sure why.

About an hour into our study time, I noticed that my left foot seemed to jump occasionally for no real reason. It was kind of like when you kick out in your sleep during some weird dream. My foot would bounce a couple of times and then settle. It probably happened four or five times over the next hour or so, but I didn't pay much attention to it. Too much caffeine can make you do strange things, so maybe that third Diet Coke of the day was not a good idea after all. Once again, though, looking back at these events with the knowledge I now have, I can see where a pattern was starting to develop. I just didn't know to look for it at the time.

The next couple of weeks passed without much fanfare. I spent hours going over my immense Quizlet index card set of terms, names, and theories until I knew all 355 cards by heart and could almost recite them backward if I had to. I was ready for the big day as comp day came calling.

It's about a forty-five-minute drive from my house to the Piedmont College campus. I put on some music and headed to meet the challenge of the day. For almost the entire duration of the trip, that crazy left-foot bounce came and went. Surely it was just nerves. What else could it possibly be? What else indeed?

Luckily, my newfound skill of impersonating Thumper did not present itself very often during the actual comps exam. There were a couple of times when I would rest my left arm on my left leg to calm the bounce down some, but those times were few and far between. The exam lasted about three hours, and by the time it was over, my brain was officially drained of all relevant knowledge and it was time to head home. The waiting would begin. Waiting for results of the test was nerve-racking. The waiting, however, would not be limited to finding out the score on an exam. Far from it!

CHAPTER 4

Moments of Truth

"Results"—that was all it said in the subject line of the email that came about a week later. Now in mid-August, I was about to click a single button on my computer and see what the reward was for all my studying and preparation for the comps exam. My mind was racing like a kid on Christmas morning. Racing down the stairs and ready to tear open my "present" that was so plainly wrapped in an email wrapping, I hoped for the best. A new bike? A PlayStation 5? A passing grade on my comps? It was all the same.

My overactive imagination began to take over. If the results are good, would they have just labeled the email subject line as "Results"? Wouldn't they have wanted to ease any fears that might appropriately be building in the minds of the email recipients? Shouldn't they say "Congratulations" in the subject line to allay the worries that were sure to be mounting? That would be the nice thing to do instead of hanging us all out like this on a shaky branch of uncertainty and wonder! What if it's bad news? If that were true, the "Results" word would make more sense. One might not know what to expect if that was the label. It could go either way—good or bad.

Enough already! Just open the email!

Then it hit me. I had forgotten one of the basic rules of email communication: read the "From" line to see who is sending you such important news as the results of something! Had I done that, I could have saved myself the quizzical expression that was surely on my face when I looked at the text of the email and did not see the clearly defined prestigious green lion that was the mascot of Piedmont College. Instead, the main heading and the footer of the document featured another title that, had I thought about it much at all, might have brought an equal degree of concern and anxiety to me. It read, "Gwinnett Rehab Clinic."

"What?"

Of course! I had forgotten all about the last visit I had at the physical therapy facility. The same nurse who had given me the grand tour and released the army of red wasps upon my shoulder was contacting me to tell me that she was satisfied with the progress I had made in my visits with her and that she was recommending no more follow-up visits. Of course, she reminded me that if things got worse, I could always return for more sessions, but I would have to get it approved through my insurance first. Funny how such a simple item as a label on an email can cause such a disruption. Maybe it was the stress of the entire situation just playing tricks with me and messing with my head. Maybe, though, it was just another step in the precarious journey down this challenging road.

*****

It was only a couple of days later as my birthday month of August began to reach its waning stages that more results found their way to my inbox. There was not as much of a shroud of mystery and suspense with this one as when the confusing rehab results email was sent. This one clearly stated "Comps Results" on the subject line, so I knew to prepare myself for the news from the Piedmont College graduate school staff. If I had wanted to make it more stressful and dramatic, I probably could have, but after the rehab email experience, I had learned a thing or two. Don't get caught up in the dramatics when you don't have to. Don't make things either bigger or worse than what they actually are. Finally, don't get caught up in trying to read between the lines. Simply put, just open the email!

Within seconds, all was well...

"Congratulations! It is our pleasure to inform you that you have passed your comps exam taken recently. You are now cleared to be accepted as a dissertation candidate for your EdD. We look forward to helping you reach your goals as you prepare to finish your work at Piedmont College."

The celebration that ensued most certainly involved some loud noises and jumping movements, not caused, however, by any involuntary muscle twitches that could be distracting. This was full-blown, childlike, over-the-moon excitement and jubilation!

"Praise the Lord!" I exclaimed.

I began sending screenshots of the acceptance news to anyone and everyone I could think of. I wanted the world to know that I was one step closer to a degree. I was one step closer to completing a challenge that, at times, seemed unattainable. Don't forget… I was also one step closer to joining "the club." Just one step away! There's an interesting line in one of the Indiana Jones movies as another quest for some historical relic is underway that has that same sentiment of being just one step away. It's at this point where the astute archaeologist and hero explains to his partner, "That's usually where the floor goes out from under you." I might not, at this point of my life's journey, have been looking for the Holy Grail, the Ark of the Covenant, or some other treasure in the sand. But what I was looking for was just as valuable. I was searching for closure to all these crazy scenarios in my world. I was ready for things to get back to some semblance of "normal."

*****

August was now behind me, and I rolled right into a rambunctious month of September 2016. I had managed to do something that all teachers pray for as school begins in August—survive the first month! It wasn't easy, but I had struggled, scratched, and clawed my way through the first six weeks and was now settling in to the "routine" of a high school teacher. I had been hoping for "normal," but sometimes you have to be careful what you hope for because you might just get it. I certainly did!

The sophomore essays were trickling in, even though, at times, it seemed more like a series of crashing waves on the shoreline that was my office desk. There were supervision duties to take care of, tests to write and to grade, class periods to teach, and lesson plans to create and revise, and there were football games to attend at the end of a crazy week of school. Yes, all was "normal" again in my world. School was in session, I had ample time to complain about how busy and tired I always was, and I was back in the offices and hallways surrounded by amazing students and incredible colleagues who were all working together to make the best of all the chaos and craziness that was the opening grading period of the 2016–2017 school year. The problem with being in a normal state, though, is that you tend not to remain there for as long a period as you would like. Something always comes along to shake the branches on which you are precariously perched. Now, I guess, it was just my turn to be ruffled up a bit.

On September 23, 2016, my "normal" began to sway. I was in the middle of grading some papers, and as I reached for the next stack to move from one side of my desk to the other, it happened again—my left shoulder and arm were on fire! School was over for the day. Good thing! Not many people were around to hear my groaning and complaining. My doctors had told me that if anything like this happened "down the road" to reach out to my chiropractor and go back in for some rehab and recovery visits. Dr. Randy, here I come! Mangle me. Manipulate me. Whatever it takes, I am "all in" to make this go away. The pain that I thought I had conquered was now trying to reclaim its territory and was doing a fine job in that effort.

Three days later (and what seemed much longer than the seventy-two hours it actually was), I was back on the "mangling mat" and ready for recovery to begin. Dr. Randy went through the normal initial observations and checkpoints and then positioned me facedown, as usual, on the table. Knowing a bit more about how this all works, I was expecting the traditional "Just relax" command—otherwise known in chiropractic circles as the green flag to begin the torture and "manipulation" of the patient. Something else, though, took its place...

"How long has this been happening?"

"The shoulder? Just a couple of days, but it's been pretty intense."

"No, not the shoulder... Your left foot is bouncing quite a bit."

"Yeah. It happens from time to time over the past couple of months, but I think it's just nerves or something."

"It's the 'or something' that has me a bit concerned."

Dr. Randy then proceeded to tell me the reason for his concerns. He said that while he was not qualified to offer an "official" diagnosis based on his observations, he did feel obliged to alert me that he had seen responses like this before, and they needed to be checked out by a specialist fairly soon. After a brief conversation, Dr. Randy agreed to submit a referral to a local neurologist he knew through the Gwinnett Clinic. Not only was this neurologist, Dr. Dinesh Raju, a specialist in Parkinson's but he was also local and accepting new patients.

While Dr. Randy went down the hallway to make the arrangements with Dr. Raju, I began to make my own analysis of this rapidly changing situation. At first, my level of concern was low. Surely, I thought, this was nothing to be worried about. I had been through the physical therapy portion of the shoulder injury, and they had warned me that there could be some repeating episodes down the line. They had even told me what to do about it if the pain returned. I was doing just what they had told me to do. What could possibly go wrong?

Of course, the other part of my brain was running wild with mysterious and ominous scenarios. I tried to process why the "injury" was now manifesting itself in a different manner but could not arrive at a viable solution or diagnosis. What was the connection between my left shoulder and a possible pinched nerve and the jumping of my left foot? I'm no medical expert (the understatement of the century), but it seems a bit far-fetched for the two extremities to be connected. I guess this is why I was back here in Dr. Randy's office trying to get some answers. If it was answers I was seeking, they were about to begin arriving.

As usual, there was good news and there was bad news. I think those items are eternally linked together when it comes to times like these. On the "bad" side of the ledger, Dr. Randy told me that Dr. Raju was adamant about seeing me right away. That couldn't be a good prognosis, but maybe he was acting out of an abundance of caution. It's kind of like the mechanic calling you and asking if you can bring your car to his shop immediately and that you "probably shouldn't be driving it right now." Really? How was I supposed to get it there if I'm not supposed to be driving it? But I digress. On the "good" side, while Dr. Raju had informed Dr. Randy that it would normally take about three to four weeks for a new patient to make it through the system, he would clear a special slot on his calendar and get me in tomorrow. That's "good," right?

*****

Throughout all this medical upheaval, there was still this little matter of trying to maintain some degree of normal contact with my job. I had missed two days of work the week leading up to my visit to Dr. Randy, which led to my referral to Dr. Raju. My colleagues knew that I was out for doctor visits, and they were aware, at least to some degree, that I was having shoulder issues again, but they did not know the extent of some of my visits and even some of the results as I had been away from my classroom and off campus for a little while. The only person on campus who knew all the details was my principal, and he was solidly in my corner, reminding me to do what I needed to do to be healthy and not to worry about my school responsibilities during all these uncertain times.

I consider myself remarkably blessed to work in such an atmosphere as my current job. In my fifteen-plus years of working there, I had noticed that the faculty, staff, administration, and students were some of the most compassionate people around. It was nothing to stop and have a prayer session in the middle of a community meeting or class session for a colleague in need or a student who may be having difficult circumstances. I had been in countless settings on campus where it was obvious that the mundane task of educating children, preparing lesson plans, organizing help sessions, and performing required meetings, while important, took second billing to developing a supportive sense of community that reached beyond the walls of the school buildings and the campus perimeter.

Here I was, now the one in need. Instead of playing the role of the giver, I was trying to adjust to being in what seemed to me to be an uncomfortable and unusual role of the receiver of support from my colleagues. I faced an unexpected dilemma at this point. I needed to share details of my experiences with my colleagues, but I did not want to cause any undue alarm. What if the visit to Dr. Raju came back as nothing serious? What if it was inconclusive? I wouldn't want to have raised concerns of others when it wasn't warranted. I struggled with this issue for about an hour while staring at my computer screen and the blank email that reflected back at me waiting for the "perfect words" to be typed and sent to others.

After a bit of mental gymnastics, which featured quite a few starts and stops of introductions and opening lines that eventually got discarded, I remembered my "solution" from earlier email scenarios and tweaked it slightly…

"Just *type* the email!"

So it began—my missive statement to my English department colleagues explaining what I was experiencing and what the next twenty-four hours might hold. I detailed the latest visit to Dr. Randy and the referral to the neurologist. While not wanting to sound any alarms, I did try to get across to my colleagues that my level of concern was increasing the more time I spent thinking about the whole ordeal. I asked for prayers from the group and, of course, knew that was a given. I asked for my wife and two girls to be included as they were also a bit concerned with the whole process not being resolved sooner or with a simpler, less-challenging outcome. By the time I finished the email and sent it, I felt a bit more secure. I definitely felt a bit more relieved. I still, however, felt an uncomfortable degree of uncertainty. I guess that was normal—and "normal" is what I have been trying to access lately.

The day of my visit to Dr. Raju was also a "milestone" day on campus. It was Homecoming Week 2016 after all, and that called for a higher degree of silliness than usual with my fellow English teachers. The morning of my visit, a picture popped up on Facebook of the entire English department dressed in their favorite professional sports team's attire. There were LA Dodgers, Boston Red Sox, and

Atlanta Falcons on display. But sadly, there was no representation of the St. Louis Cardinals as I was not in attendance. I did get a "mention" in the caption that stated the group was not at full force as one of us was missing and that they sent their thoughts and prayers in my direction.

I had actually forgotten that it was homecoming week with all this other stuff going on in my life. At least, if I had to miss several days of class due to a medical issue, this was probably not a bad week for it to happen. Let's just say that not a lot of serious academic work gets done during Homecoming Week, so I wasn't going to be terribly behind when I returned. The homecoming football game was going to be the next day, and I hoped that I would be able to celebrate my own type of "homecoming" that day, as well as I could return to work with great news and life could slowly find its old lane again and I could steer myself back into my routines. If only it were that simple.

*****

That September 2016 morning was especially nice. The fall season was just kicking in, and the morning was crisp, but not freezing. If only I felt as comfortable as the weather that morning. My wife, Becky, had taken off work so that she could accompany me to the appointment. We had discussed whether or not she should go to this appointment, but she felt the need to be there so that she could hear any important information firsthand. She knew that sometimes I was not the world's greatest relayer of medical situations and scenarios. She was right. I tended to synthesize previous doctor's diagnoses and instructions down to what I thought was significant and just tell Becky about that part. Often, though, I would leave out some significant piece of information that was actually quite critical to the whole process. She did not want to leave this appointment up to chance or to my analytical tendencies or mental recall. That's a good thing!

While in the waiting room, my wife and I had the usual nervous conversation one would expect at a time like this. Each of us might have secretly had our own conclusions about the potential outcome of this visit, but we kept the spoken part of our concerns to the perfunctory concepts of "I'm sure this is all going to work out" and "No matter what, the doctor will know what to do." I thought I would be even more nervous in the waiting room, but I tried my best to remain calm and logical about the whole ordeal. My logical side was trying to reassure my emotional side that there was bound to be a reasonable cause for the issue with my shoulder and my bouncing foot. Reasonable causes, I deduced, usually come with reasonable solutions. At least, I thought that was how it should work.

After a relatively short wait in the lobby, I was called back to meet with Dr. Raju. My first impression was that he seemed to be a rather knowledgeable doctor and that he was genuinely concerned with trying to figure out what was going on in my medical world. This was a relief as I have been to doctors before and thought that I was just another person on the list, just another appointment to be met and completed, and have left appointments not knowing any more than I did when I arrived. Using my previous mechanic's analogy, it would be like waiting all afternoon at the repair shop while your car is being worked on, and then after being given the final diagnosis and completing the required work, you pay your bill and hop in your car to go home. However, as you approach the first intersection away from the repair shop, the red check engine light comes on, you hear a strangely metallic-sounding groan, and you come coasting to a stop on the side of the road. Bummer!

Following a brief conversation about the events leading up to the visit, Dr. Raju told me that he was going to have me go through some routine exercises so that he could evaluate my movements and see what was going on. I never realized that clinching my left fist while rotating my right arm in big circles would be so difficult or so telling. I repeated the fist-and-arm exercise on the opposite side and found it a bit easier but still more challenging than I expected. We proceeded to the standard reflexology test with the rubber mallet on each knee, and then I was instructed to kick out with each leg, one at a time, against some mild resistance to test my leg strength and amount of mobility. It was during this portion of the examination routine that my left foot bounced a bit for the first time during the visit, bringing about some concern on my part and an obvious note-taking opportunity for the doctor.

As the procedure moved forward, my arm strength, grip strength, and vision tracking were also evaluated. With each passing portion of the testing, I grew less and less certain of whether or not I was producing the "right" results. Of course, what did I know what should be "right" and what should be "wrong"? I was just a confused patient looking for some answers so that I could begin a course of action and/or treatment that would bring my life back to normal again. There's that word again—*normal.* My current definition of that word was about to change drastically in the next few minutes.

What turned out to be the final portions of the evaluation took place in the hallway outside of my assigned examination room. Dr. Raju had me walk several yards away from him, turn, and then return. This was done three times as notes were taken and opinions were drawn, which would soon be revealed. Finally, the doctor had me stand directly in front of him, facing away, with my arms folded across my chest. He told me to just relax as he tugged slightly on my shoulders in an attempt to pull me back toward him. The first two times, I staggered a bit and took a small step toward the doctor. On the third and final tug, that step was a bit more pronounced. Once again, I wondered what it all meant. Was I doing it right? Were the results promising? The time for answers was drawing near.

As Dr. Raju guided me back into the examination room, he told me that he was going to look over all the results, consult with some-one on his team, and then come back in and tell me what he found. Now it was just my wife and I alone with only a short amount of time standing between us and the outcome of these past few months of trying times. Becky is my rock in times like these. Always has been. Always will be. While she does have her emotional moments, she also has the uncanny ability to remain calm in some of the most difficult circumstances. While I struggle along and fumble trying to figure out what to do or say next in a tight spot, Becky always comes through and asks the questions that I forgot to pose. She processes information with a greater balance of reality than I do. She doesn't accept everything at face value. Instead, she wants to get through all the extraneous baggage in a situation and find a way to cut to the chase and get to the bottom line. I love her for that because it's a skill that I'm still trying to develop (and not succeeding too frequently I might add). It's crazy to me now that we even questioned whether or not she should come along for this appointment. Only an insane fool would want to go do it alone in a critical moment like this regardless of the outcome. If it were great news, there would be someone right there to celebrate with. If there was uncertainty, she would automatically know what to say next as a follow-up to get to the bottom of it. If it were a serious result, she would be there to help me process it all and have just the right thing to say. Moments later, the door opened, and after a brief explanation of what he was looking for and what he actually observed, Dr. Raju said those fateful words, "You have early onset Parkinson's."

There it was! On the day before the homecoming football game, any thoughts of good times and celebrations on campus were replaced with shock and disbelief. Of all the possible outcomes that I had been reading up on since my chiropractic visit that led to this referral, this was the one I was hoping not to hear. Surely he's made a mistake. Parkinson's is an "old person" disease. I'm only forty-eight. That's not old! What happened to the "pinched nerve theory" or the "rotator cuff impairment" possibilities? What happens now? The crazy, illogical side of my brain even dared to wonder how much time I had left. It was all coming too fast!

Dr. Raju went on to explain that I was actually the third-youngest Parkinson's patient whom he was observing and treating at the time. Well, at least there was that! I'm part of a "record" or something! Silencing my sarcastic self a bit, I continued listening to the diagnosis and the treatment plan.

Instead of simply rushing headlong into a standardized regimen of meds that just any Parkinson's patient might be prescribed, Dr. Raju explained his plan this way. He wanted to get a better grasp of exactly what impact my disease was having on my work in the classroom. Knowing that, he could then figure out the right type and dosage of medications that would serve my schedule the best while working to maintain as high a quality of life as possible. That was one of the most reassuring statements I heard all day. Dr. Raju stepped forward in my book with that remark as it became clearer that this was not going to be a standard "Take two of these and call me in the morning" approach to care. Instead, Dr. Raju wanted to personalize the treatment and get me the highest quality of results possible.

Before any medications would be prescribed, I had homework. For the next few weeks, I was assigned to keep two logs. First, I would keep a tabulation of how many times each hour I experienced a noticeable tremor. Second, I would track my sleep hours each night and then rate the previous night's sleep on a scale when I got up each morning. If anything out of the ordinary occurred—like crazy dreams, kicking out in my sleep, cramping, or talking in my sleep—I would make a note of that also. As someone fascinated with statistics and numbers, this seemed not only doable but also interesting to me. Anything I could do to gather the best information needed was fine by me.

With my homework assigned, Dr. Raju could tell that Becky and I were still in the processing stage of all this. He said that he would give me a copy of the instructions on the way out of the office. More than that, though, he told us to stay in the examination room as long as we needed, to talk things over, and when we were ready, to come find him to check out. With that, the doctor who had just told me (in so many words) that my life was about to drastically change walked out.

It didn't take long. I turned to Becky, knowing that she would have the right thing to say at this crazy moment. She did! It was nothing! She just hugged me tight and let me get it all out of my system. Tears were plentiful for both of us for the next few minutes as we both realized that things were different now. Still, though, even with the diagnosis and all the changes that were coming in our lives over the next few weeks, months, and years, some things remained the same. My wife still loves me. I have the greatest two kids in the world. I have colleagues who care about me. Most importantly, I have a god that will not put me through things I cannot bear. It was going to be okay. Different, but okay. We gathered ourselves a bit, tried to make our eyes a little less red, and left the examination room, entering the next stage of the journey hand in hand.

PART 2
The Life Lessons

CHAPTER 5

Life Lesson 1—Mind over Matter

Most of us would agree it is best to go through life as a continual learner. Agreeing with that sentiment, though, does not make the desire to accomplish the said goal any stronger or make the pathway to the finish line of becoming a lifelong learner any shorter or easier to navigate. Still, if one focuses on making themselves better by increasing their knowledge, odds are they will spend more time using that knowledge to assist others while also improving their own experience. Such is the situation in which I have found myself as I deal with Parkinson's.

I have dedicated countless hours to watching videos on the life of a Parkinson's patient. I've seen the stories of those who have endured or are considering the invasive deep brain stimulation surgery designed to alleviate the tremors that plague most, if not all, Parkinson's patients. I have read both of Michael J. Fox's books written from the celebrity perspective of having Parkinson's. I've studied and contributed to the National Parkinson's Foundation as well as the Michael J. Fox Foundation. In short, I feel I know a good bit about the disease, its trademark symptoms, its progression, and its outcomes. However, while I have gained a significant amount of information, these facts, figures, testimonials, and studies are not the most important source of my learning as a Parkinson's patient. The most impactful education takes place "between the lines" and "on the field of play" that demarcates my everyday existence. Put another way, I have learned a great deal *about* Parkinson's, but I feel I have learned even more *from* Parkinson's and my day-to-day life.

In my classroom, I constantly stress to my students the importance of learning by doing. Sure, someone can study all the grammar books they want and review writing style guidelines until they are blue in the face, but the real education in the writing experience comes when you put pencil to paper or fingers to the keyboard and start producing content. The same applies to a Parkinson's patient. Reading up on the disease and the impacts on someone's life is one thing. It's entirely something else when a Parkinson's patient realizes and appreciates the variety and significance of the lessons confronting them each and every time they get up in the morning. If it's true that experience is the best teacher, then a Parkinson's patient's life experience is a challenging taskmaster. It is my hope that by sharing some of my experiences and lessons I have learned in the last few years, I can bring hope to other Parkinson's patients while also reminding myself that there is still plenty to learn on this journey. It's all about putting mind over matter!

*****

After the initial diagnosis from Dr. Raju and the homework assigned to me to begin recording important data on a regular basis, I knew that I was in for a challenge. What exactly do I record? How accurate does the information need to be? What if it's not perfect? I had to figure out a system—and fast—if this was going to work and be something of value to the doctor and his team. This was going to require some thought and some planning if it is going to work. However, before any of that planning could take place, there was the small matter of going to work tomorrow and facing the real world again.

I had been out of work for a couple of days while going through the appointments and testing, and I had to make a decision about my reentry. It was not a decision I was ready to make. I called my principal and had a heart-to-heart conversation about my progress, the official diagnosis, and forecast for my condition. What I thought might be a difficult call turned out to be a rich blessing for me. After speaking with my boss, I was reassured that my school was ready to support me 100 percent and do whatever was needed to make this work as my condition progressed. Deep down, I have always "known" that my colleagues are amazing and caring people. I've seen them in action in my years of employment, and I know what they are capable of doing. I've seen meals arranged, visits made, cards and letters written from the heart, and a million other awesome acts of kindness performed by people who can only be described as God's right-hand folks. Now it was my turn to be on the receiving end of their kindness and support.

Still in a bit of shock over the whole diagnosis process and the results, I was not quite ready to face the crowd at work just yet, so I chose to take the next day off to wrap my head around the whole thing and try to prepare myself for what was to come on Monday. This would also give me time to talk with my wife some more and also break the news to my two girls before returning to work. I didn't really know how much I expected to figure out over a three-day weekend, but at least I would not have to tell my story and explain my situation over and over again to my colleagues just yet. I would have time to prepare for that over the weekend break.

In an effort to get ahead of things a bit, I sat down at my computer and sent a detailed email to my English department colleagues on Thursday night. In it, I revealed my diagnosis and current medical treatment plans. I asked for prayers from the group and hoped they would include my daughters in those prayers as I prepared to break the news to them over the weekend. I was not sure how that was going to go, so praying for some wisdom and simply the correct words to say to explain the situation to them was definitely in the cards. Within just a few minutes of sending the email, the responses started flowing in. As expected, the comments were supportive and compassionate while also tinged with a bit of disbelief and shock. I could relate to those feelings all too well. They were getting to be the norm for me lately.

That night, I sat down with my family and worked up the courage to explain to my daughters what was going on and what it all meant. I think I might have used a phrase like "I'm not dying from this" too many times, but it seemed reassuring in the moment. I am not 100 percent certain how much my teenage daughters comprehended of all the medical information I threw their way in what ended up being a much shorter family meeting than I expected. They had a fair number of questions, and on the surface, they seemed to handle it quite well. I, on the other hand, was a nervous wreck during the whole process! I never thought I'd be having such a serious medical conversation with my daughter at their age or, for that matter, my age. Still, we got through it and prepared ourselves for what was certain to be a rapidly changing future. We agreed that no matter what comes along, we had one another and our faith in God Almighty, and that would surely be enough.

*****

"I can do this," I said to myself as I was sitting in my car in the faculty parking lot with my coffee and breakfast in hand. This was my attempt to ready myself for the first day back to reality as I went back to work following my diagnosis. A little self-talk couldn't hurt. I don't think what I was feeling is best categorized as "fear" as it was a limited level of confidence. Deep inside, I knew what was going to happen. There would be hugs and well-wishes from colleagues and plenty of questions from everyone. My students, not yet aware of the circumstances of my extended absence, would be curious about why I had been away and would want to be included in the process. I was certain they could handle the information. I would have to fill them in as I would be tracking my daily tremor activity on my phone while in class. That record keeping started immediately, but I still wasn't sure of what the numbers would reveal. Maybe when I had gone a week or two down the road and had a larger sample size of data, I would have a clearer picture of what this was going to be like in the long run.

In order to keep better records of my tremor activity, I made a spreadsheet broken down into the hours of the day. I kept it handy on my phone and my classroom iPad so that I could record the information easily and without causing too big of a distraction while teaching. The instructions were fairly simple. Each time I noticed that my tremors were "activated," I would make a tally mark or note on my spreadsheet. The activity would be broken down by each hour of the day so that my doctor could try to discover any behavioral patterns involved in my tremor activity. Dr. Raju had told me that some younger Parkinson's patients have a distinct "on-and-off period" pattern that could be initially managed with a specific dosage and routine of medications. His hope was such a pattern could be identified in the four to six weeks of information I would be collecting.

In a way, I felt like Pavlov's dog. My leg or arm would twitch, and I would instinctively reach for my device and record the event. Maybe fifteen minutes later, the process would repeat itself. I'm sure my students were wondering what was going on for the first couple of days as I kept my phone and iPad on the desk more than usual and went back and forth from it many more times than usual. Soon, I knew I would have to include them in the process. It was the safe thing to do in case there was ever a rare Parkinson's medical emergency in the classroom. It was also the right thing to do.

After a few days of recording the information, the time had come for me to tell my students what was going on. It was a Friday, so I would see all my classes in the same day instead of having them split into two groups on a block day schedule. As when I broke the news to my colleagues, part of me knew how this was going to go, but another part of me wasn't quite sure. I felt certain the majority of my students would be mature enough to handle the information. They would be supportive and genuinely concerned and would want to do what they could to help. I wasn't as sure about a small group of my students who were either not as involved in any aspect of school to be concerned with what their English teacher was going through or did not think it cool to be vulnerable enough to show compassion in a group setting. I couldn't worry about those few, if any, students who might not be in a good enough place to handle the information. I just had to lay it all on the table and see what would happen.

As a precaution, I emailed all my students' parents on the morning I was going to reveal my condition and diagnosis to the classes. I let them know what was going on so that they would not be caught off guard by their children that afternoon bombarding them with only parts of the story that might cause some undue stress and concern. I did not want one of my students to hop in their mom's car that afternoon and boldly exclaim that their English teacher was dying! That would not go over well. Before I could even get to my first class, my email inbox was filling up with amazing notes of concern, compassion, and support from the parents. I even discovered a few of them had experience with Parkinson's in their immediate family. It was a good start to a good day.

Each class period had basically the same reaction to the news. They had lots of questions and wanted to know how they could help. I reassured them that I was still in the initial stages of gathering information for my doctor and that I would know more in the upcoming weeks. My eleventh-grade students even stopped the class after I had explained it all to them. Led by one of the class leaders, they huddled up around me and offered an amazing prayer of support and concern. That was the highlight of the day!

"They get it! They really get it!"

*****

One's attitude plays a vital role in the degree of success one has in life. It's all too easy to find yourself doubting the fairness of any situation in which you are placed. Countless amounts of energy can be wasted by focusing on things we cannot change or by worrying about things that are beyond our control. We all know that remaining positive is the better way to live, but we don't often want to invest the time it takes to adjust our ways of thinking in order to maintain a positive outlook. Such was my case in the early stages of my Parkinson's journey. If I didn't remind myself to try to be positive, it would become inevitable that I would backtrack into a world of negativity, stress, and worry that would be counterproductive to trying to be an effective educator. My students noticed it. My colleagues noticed it. My family noticed it. It just took longer than it should before I noticed it. This is not to say I conquered it every single day. Nothing could be further from the truth. It was (and still is) a constant battle in which I have to train myself not to be afraid to take the more difficult mental path toward positivity. My first steps down that path came with the introduction of my first Parkinson's medications.

After recording my tremor activity and tracking my sleep through various apps for most of October and November, I returned to Dr. Raju's office in the month of December for my follow-up visit. Armed with a notebook filled with numbers, facts, and observations, I was optimistic. I felt like a proud student who had gone above and beyond the call of duty in doing their homework, and I was ready to present my work to the class. Surely the teacher would be impressed with all my labors.

Dr. Raju did appreciate all the time and effort I had put forth to collect the information he needed. We discussed the information I had gathered by focusing on my observations of how I was managing at the daily tasks of being a high school teacher. Dr. Raju wanted to know the extent of the impact the tremors and other Parkinson's symptoms were having on my daily life and routine.

"How close to your normal self do you feel lately?"

I had to stop and think about that one for a moment. That *N* word had just shown up again. My honest answer to that question was, "Not at all." Instead of focusing on lesson plans, quiz scores, classroom management, and the all-important early morning coffee routine I have, I was delegating time to thinking about and recording tremors and wondering how much the students really noticed my hand, arm, or leg jumping from time to time. Normal? Not so much. Unique and challenging? Most definitely.

After a discussion of the information I had collected, Dr. Raju put me through an abbreviated version of the mobility tests that had been performed on my day of diagnosis. Following that, the prescription of my first series of medication was explained. I was going to be given a medicine known in the market as Sinemet. It is a basic combination of carbidopa and levodopa that is a standard-issue drug for Parkinson's patients. The key lies in the proper dosage of the prescription. Too little of one-half of the medication and there is basically no impact on the patient at all. Too much and, to put it in the words of the doctor, you will know it pretty quickly. I'll just let your mind wander and come to your own disgusting conclusions on that one.

As with any new medication, my concern was with potential side effects. Dr. Raju was very open about the potential impacts, and they did not seem too bad at first. He detailed some jittery feelings that sometimes come with the correct dosage and maybe some sleeping issues in some people, though the chances of that were not great with someone my age. Okay, these are things I can handle. Let's do this. Then there was the last little detail of potential nausea that was a fairly common side effect of the medication. I knew there was a catch, and this was it! I am easily defined as what is known as a character of "weak constitution." Simply put, if there is even a microscopic chance that something may cause nausea, it is a guaranteed certainty that I will experience it. I am also known to be a very lousy patient when it comes to (as the doctor called it once during my visit) "gastrointestinal distress." Anyone who has ever been around me in times of stomach bugs, food poisoning, or other pleasant events of such nature can attest to the fact that one might think I was dying in the said moments of "gastrointestinal distress." Indeed, there have probably been some people—my wife included—who have even considered helping me toward my goal of looming death in times such as these. I think you get the picture!

Even with my "gastric concerns," Dr. Raju convinced me that this medication was the proper choice for me at my current stage of the disease's progression. He noted that since my tremor logs showed what he deemed to be "low" to "mild" tremor activity, he was only prescribing the lowest possible dosage to begin with. I would stay on this regimen of meds for a couple of months, and then he would reevaluate the dosage in my next follow-up visit. In the meantime, it would be important for me to continue to track tremor activity as I start the new prescription. This would give the doctors the clearest picture of the effectiveness of the medication. My thoughts? "Here goes nothing!"

I believe the words Dr. Raju used to describe the potential for nausea with the medication as "a fairly common side effect." Truer words have never been spoken! I started the Sinemet in mid-December and got a firsthand look at the so-called fairly common side effects pretty quickly. *Nausea* was the word of the day for the first couple of weeks of the treatment. Originally, I had considered waiting to start the meds over the upcoming Christmas break from school, but I decided I wanted to get the initiation period over with, so I started about a week before the break. Bad move! I had been used to counting and recording my tremor activity on my phone for the past couple of months. Now it would have been more appropriate (though quite disgusting) to keep a record of the times I felt like I was going to hurl so badly that one of my lungs might come up. I probably shouldn't paint such an awful picture of this time in the treatment process. By no means was I in such bad shape that I was living in the restroom (though, at times, the thought did cross my mind). Remember how I stated earlier that I am not a good patient when in the throes of nausea? Bad patients tend to exaggerate how awful they feel at any given time. Enough said.

December turned to January, and the time continued to roll along fairly quickly as I approached my late February follow-up visit with Dr. Raju. I looked forward to telling him about the "pleasures" of handling the side effects in my world, but I was also more and more curious about the impacts of the medication when compared to my tremor logs from the previous months. In my own nonmedical opinion, I wasn't seeing an enormous impact on the number of the intensity of the tremors. Life seemed pretty much the same as it was at the start of the prescription, and that was getting to be a source of frustration. I guess I didn't really quite know what I expected out of all this. Did I honestly think that taking a pill in the morning and another in the afternoon would be enough to totally wipe out this disease? In my mind, I knew better than that, but I guess the thought that a miracle could occur was still there. This was another test of my ability to find the positive side of my daily routine. No, two pills a day would not be a cure. There is no cure for this disease yet. But by reminding myself that I was on a continual journey toward getting better and the goal was to maintain the quality of my everyday existence, it was a bit easier to look for the silver lining in the storm clouds that swirled around me, even if I had to constantly ask myself where the nearest bathroom was…just in case!

*****

In the early stages of my Parkinson's journey, many people in my circle suggested I keep myself busy in order to decrease the likelihood of me sitting around focusing on my condition and feeling sorry for myself. An active mind, these friends reminded me, would help me keep a more upbeat outlook on life in general and serve as a frontline attack to ward off any episodes of depression or excess worry. Keeping my mind busy was not going to be a problem at this point as I was fully engaged in completing my doctoral dissertation. If anything could serve as a mental distraction, working on a two-hundred-page document that reflected the last eighteen months of intensive study and research should do the trick.

Having completed the doctoral comprehensive exams in August before my diagnosis, I had moved onto the next portion of my study. The classes I was scheduled to attend were mostly brainstorming and planning sessions designed to get the creative juices flowing and provide some organization, analysis, and feedback on my work. If that did not keep me mentally engaged, then I don't know what else would. However, there was still the matter of having to deal with the physical issues involved in my Parkinson's lifestyle. Tremors during classes could be a problem. At least there was not an enormous number of classes I had to attend in the months of September and October of 2016—the two months leading up to my diagnosis. If there were going to be any medical issues during this time, the social impacts of being in a classroom with my cohort members would be limited.

The last class meeting in October proved to be a blessing in disguise and a boost to my positive outlook. That evening's class was a three-hour ordeal in which we would present our sketches of our dissertations to the group and, for the first time, have to publicly describe our research intentions. After working for days to get the sketch at least to a point where I could present a semi-intelligent discussion of my ideas and research processes, I walked into the class-room with a higher level of confidence than I expected. Numbers were drawn for the order of presentations, and I got number 3. As soon as our professor had given us our final instructions and announced the first presenter, it happened! Tremors in my left foot struck with full force! I literally had to hold my leg down with my left hand to keep it in some degree of stability. At first, I was not too overly con-cerned about the ordeal. Based on my observations, I knew that it would pass soon and all would be well. Something was different this time though. While I had informed my colleagues at work and the students in my classes about my diagnosis in the recent weeks, the members of my doctoral cohort did not know what had transpired in my life in this critical month of October 2016.

David Sells, one of my closest friends and frequent research partner in the cohort, was sitting next to me when the bouncing started. He looked over and wanted to be sure everything was okay. I assured him that it was and that I would fill him in later on. I had been debating for a couple of weeks whether or not to reveal my diagnosis to the cohort class and my professors. I did not want to become a sympathy case who gets passed along in the doctoral pro-cess because someone felt sorry for me and wanted to see me succeed. I also did not want to fall into the mental trap of using my diagnosis as a crutch and an excuse for not doing my best work in this critical academic portion of my professional career. If I was going to gain membership into my family's "doctoral club," it was going to be on my own merit and not because someone had given me something I did not deserve in the process.

The first two presentations had been completed, and it was now my turn to take the stand. The tremors in my left foot had subsided, and all things seemed normal again. There it was. Normal? I should have known better! My presentation began very strongly. I was detail-ing my research questions and the methodology I was planning on using to answer the questions when it happened. My left hand began to shake a bit, and I nearly dropped the remote presentation clicker in my hand. It wasn't enough to throw me completely off my game, but it did distract me momentarily, and it caught David's eye as well. I guess an explanation was going to be in order for him as well as the professor if she had noticed the slight babble in the presentation. Known for her keen observation skills and bluntness in critique, my professor had surely noticed it. Now the question was if she would call me out on it in a public manner or wait to see me after the class had ended. Luckily for me, it was the latter.

My professor came over to my table after class and asked if everything was all right. My first reaction was that was a loaded question. Everything was not all right in my world. Not even close. I had learned just a few weeks ago that I had a disease with no cure, and I was right in the middle of a critical time in my journey through graduate school as well. Things were not all right! Still, though, I knew that I wanted to maintain a strong front. In response to her question, I told her that I was just experiencing a bit of nerves and that all was going to be fine. I was hoping she would buy that answer. No luck!

"I've seen too many of your presentations to believe that it was nerves. What's really going on?"

David was still there, so I figured this was the opportune time to let them both know what was going on. For the next few minutes, I laid out the events of the past few weeks before them, and they took it all in with great patience. I only saw one extra quizzical look on David's face as he listened to the explanation. In just a few short minutes, it was done. It was all out there for my graduate school world to see. What hadn't appeared yet was their reaction to the revelation.

My professor started first. "Do you remember what you heard at orientation way back when?"

It had been a while, but I said that I did. How could I possibly forget the first day of grad school?

"We told you," the professor continued, "that some of you would have life happen to you along the way to completing the program and that how those students handle life will determine how successful you will be."

She was right. Life had happened to me…and then some! I knew, though, that she was also right about it being up to me how it was going to be handled. For the last few years, I had set my sights on earning my doctorate. Maybe it was just to be able to say I was a member of "the club." Maybe it was something more. Maybe I had to prove to myself I could do it…no matter what. Parkinson's was just another curveball I had to learn how to hit. In some ways, it made me even more determined than ever to succeed. Other people may fail and not survive graduate school. I was not going to be one of them!

For the next twenty months, life was a whirlwind as May 2018 arrived—graduate school conference calls and Skype sessions with my adviser, a full load of classes jammed full of eager teenagers wanting to do anything but write essays and analyze literature, twin daughters growing up way too fast and getting closer to the end of their high school careers, draft after draft after antagonizing draft of a dissertation to fill whatever "free" time might try to pry itself into my calendar. Stress, thy name is *life*, and it was coming at me head-on with very little to slow it down prior to impact.

Even my medication routine changed a bit as Dr. Raju introduced me to a patch that was supposed to deliver a steady flow of similar medication to that found in Sinemet but with a reduced level of nausea as a side effect. Say no more! I am in! One patch was good for twenty-four hours, so I did not have to worry about taking food or counting pills or trying not to forget to take the pills in the first place. All I had to figure out was how to prepare for my dissertation defense that was supposed to happen at the end of the summer break. In some ways, I was simply living the life of a normal doctoral student.

I did it again, didn't I? Used the word *normal* again! Nothing challenges one's attempts to remain positive in the face of crazy times more than thinking you have everything figured out. When you get to that point, there is only one thing that can happen: you find out very quickly that you do not have control and you do not have everything figured out. In fact, you usually discover that you do not have a single thing figured out at all, much less the entire picture. That film is still left undeveloped in the darkroom.

The patch seemed to be working pretty well. Tremors were fewer and farther between major episodes. I would still occasionally pull out my best Thumper impersonation again and tap my foot to the rhythm of some invisible drummer. In fact, that drummer was working on increasing the tempo from time to time in an effort to create a rumba beat in my brain. It was unsettling, to say the least, but I knew that it was just part of the game. I didn't have to like the rules of the game; I simply had to accept them and learn to play by them. Of course, I could complain about the rules being unfair, but that would do no good. I knew this going in, but at least I felt a bit better when I was able to vent some of my frustrations at the way the game was progressing.

The summer ended, and my anticipated defense date got delayed just a bit. The target date was now mid-September, so I was just weeks away from defending my dissertation to a room full of academic experts who would have the final say on the status of my membership into "the club." I spoke with Dr. Raju briefly about a week before my defense date, and he assured me that my current medical allotment was going to get me through the stress of that date. I needed to hear that because my mind was already racing about the gruesome possibilities of what could happen if things went haywire on defense day. I could see myself turning an unusual shade of green as the nausea took over my entire body as I stepped behind the podium. After a feeble collection of opening remarks, the contents of my well-balanced breakfast of waffles and bacon were being spewed upon those gathered around the table. The only doctor that would be coming out of the conference room in that scenario would be the paramedic wheeling me out on a stretcher after I collapsed in a tragic heap on the floor. This was not only a test of my nerve but also a test of the level of confidence I had in my treatment and the ability to remain positive in the face of what was certain to be one of the more stressful situations I had ever faced.

All things considered, the defense presentation went well. I only caught myself having to grip the edge of the podium once or twice to fight off a tremor from taking over my left arm and hand. There were no Thumper-like foot or leg bouncing incidents. That was a relief. Before I knew it, I had finished the presentation, answered a slew of questions, and retired to the hallway to await the decision of the committee. About fifteen to twenty minutes later, the committee called me back into the conference room and congratulated me on finishing the program and earning my doctorate!

To say I was relieved at that point would be a tragic understatement. Almost three years of classes, tests, essays, research, presentations, and writing had brought me to this point. I was in "the club" now, and the celebrations could begin. Throughout this academic journey, my wife had always reminded me that I would get this done because I tend to give things 110 percent until they are done. Yes, I know that 110 percent is a mathematical impossibility, but my doctorate is in education and not mathematics! This success and my wife's words were also a reminder to me that I don't have to let Parkinson's control me. I can still live a great and fulfilling life even if I have a medical issue. Truthfully, though, at this point in my Parkinson's journey, I had not been doing a great job at that. Too many times, I found myself giving in to the symptoms, the side effects, and the lethargy that appeared at various times and drained my days. Today's defense presentation was a success, but I also realized that it was a small step in a longer journey. You don't win a marathon by being in first place at mile marker 1. You win by being the steadiest, most determined, and best-conditioned athlete in the pack. Today, I passed mile marker 1, but I was still way back in the pack even if it felt amazing and oh-so satisfying to have one mile under my belt. Of course, that just means that I have twenty-five more miles of challenges directly in front of me if I want to cross the line.

*****

Any Parkinson's patient will tell you that one of the most impactful activities you can do to help fight the progression of the disease is to stay active. It is so important to just keep moving! In the early stages of my journey, I read articles about seventy-year-old men and women with Parkinson's who took up karate or boxing classes specifically designed for Parkinson's patients. Other Parkinson's patients chose swimming or cycling as their method of staying in motion. Both activities are beneficial as muscles are kept in shape, strength is developed, and balance is increased. In the first couple of months after my diagnosis, I was also looking for what my method of staying active was going to be.

I started going for walks in my neighborhood and trying to meet my Fitbit goal of ten thousand steps each day. Between moving quite a bit at work in my classroom and going for a couple of laps around the neighborhood, I was off to a pretty good start. Around late November or early December, I joined a local gym so I could use their treadmills and stay out of the really cold weather. Throughout 2017 and 2018, I would sign up for the occasional 5K or 10K race. These events were designed and scheduled to get me in just enough shape to be able to run in the Peachtree Road Race 10K on July 4 of those years. I started running in that event (the largest 10K in the world with over sixty thousand runners converging in downtown Atlanta each year) back in 2008, and I have not missed a year since. My newfound movement incentive was enough to get me to tie up the sneakers just enough to get me to the Peachtree finish line each year.

After the 2018 Peachtree Road Race, I was not happy with my finishing time in the event. I was slowing down in my "old age." The idea crossed my mind that I needed to improve my qualifying time for the race so that I could start in one of the earlier waves of the race instead of being in the middle of the mass of humanity that was running in my wave that year. Instead of being in Wave L, I wanted to be in Wave E. If I could accomplish that, I would cross the starting line about twenty minutes sooner than my current wave and the temperature would be that much cooler during the race. Don't get me wrong. I said "cool-er." There's no such thing as a "cool" Atlanta Fourth of July!

With my plan in place, I set about to run in as many qualifying races as I could between the end of the 2018 Peachtree and the cutoff for registration for the next race, which would come in January 2019. Starting on July 13, 2019, I ran in a local race called the Frozen 5K and had a decent time (for me). I knew I could do better. One race became two races, and soon it was the middle of September. I looked at my logbook where I was tracking my results and noticed I had run in nine 5K races over nine consecutive weekends. Pretty cool!

I had an appointment with Dr. Raju for my traditional follow-up procedure near the end of September, and I mentioned to him my plan for staying active. Needless to say, he was all for it. He suggested, though, to make sure that I was keeping up with my nutrition on days before the races. One concern he had was my balance. Parkinson's patients are notorious for having balance issues at some point in their progression, so he wanted me to be sure to be hydrated and well-fed the day before a run in order to limit the chances of balance being an issue. Other than that, he gave me his blessing to continue.

I continued to pile up consecutive race weekends and collect some decent times along the way. By November, I had recorded a thirty-two-minute 5K time—two minutes slower than the thirty-minute time I would need to qualify for Wave E of the next Peachtree race. The week of Thanksgiving, I made an online donation to the Michael J. Fox Foundation as a part of their fall fundraiser program. It was not a large sum of money by any amount, but it made me think about what I might be able to do to help this organization in some way.

Looking at my race log, I noticed that I had completed twenty races over the last nineteen consecutive weekends. A thought crossed my mind. What if I could use my 5K races as a way to raise money for the Fox Foundation? It seemed crazy at first, but over the next few days, it came to life. I started a Facebook group fundraiser called Streaking for Parkinson's. I would maintain my streak of consecutive weekends with a 5K race all the way out to fifty-two consecutive weekends and celebrate the yearlong streak with the race on July 4 in Wave E of the Peachtree. Things started slowly as the races continued piling up, but by the week of Christmas, I was at twenty-six races over twenty-four consecutive weekends and had met my goal of raising $1,000 in online donations. I even made a couple of running T-shirts with the group name on them and wore those on race days. It created some conversations with runners I would meet on race days and, I hope, helped bring some awareness to the cause of Parkinson's research. I even connected with two or three other runners who were Parkinson's patients and swapped stories with them. It was a fabulous way to stay moving, but it also helped me stay focused on a goal of trying to help others along the way.

Don't let me fool you. There were many times in "the Streak" that I wanted to call the whole thing off. I couldn't though. It wouldn't be right. A few races were a bit on the rainy side, and others had me freezing my shoelaces off. Some of the races in the middle of the Streak had me melting in the early summer morning sun and humidity, but I managed to get through it.

In week 38 of the Streak, bad news came out as the COVID-19 virus began to take hold in the state of Georgia. After completing forty-four races in thirty-eight consecutive weeks, I heard on the radio that the Peachtree Road Race was going to be canceled. What? They can't do that! I was disgusted with the whole thing but kept the races coming. Forty weeks. Forty-five weeks. Fifty races. Fifty-five races. In May, the announcement was released that the Peachtree Road Race was going to be rescheduled for Thanksgiving Day. That would mean having to extend my streak about another twenty weeks. With the hot weather kicking in and the race going to be a virtual-only race, I reluctantly called an end to the Streak on July 25, 2019, with the running of the Project Lifting Spirits 5K—race number 64 in the streak of fifty-four consecutive weekends of running.

Lessons? The whole journey through the Streak had some comparisons to my entire Parkinson's experience. First, it was a test in perseverance. There were some Saturday mornings when that early alarm went off where I told myself I must be insane…especially if it was raining, superhumid, or somewhere in the low twenties for a morning low. There are Parkinson's days like that. I wish I could say that I conquered all those difficult Parkinson's days in the same manner used to keep my streak going, but that would not be true. Some really tough Parkinson's days honestly kicked my butt. Some of those days, I didn't feel like I had a choice but to take the beating, but there were some (maybe more than I would like to let on) where I allowed the butt kicking to take place because I wanted to feel defeated. Those days went into the loss column for me, but they also served as reminders to try and do better on the next tough Parkinson's day that came my way. I can compare it to some of my early race times in the beginning events of the Streak. On those race days, I expected my time to be in the thirty- to thirty-two-minute range. Then something would go haywire, and I would post a thirty-nine- or forty-minute-plus time and just feel disgusted with the whole thing. Still, there was another race to get ready for in seven days, so it was a matter of finding a way to get over it and move on. Once again, some weeks I did that better than others, and some weeks I would let a bad race affect me for the next event on the calendar. That was exceptionally frustrating but difficult to avoid some weeks.

In my Parkinson's experience, the same is true. Some weeks would have one or two challenging days where I didn't sleep well (or at all) or the tremors would come after me hard and heavy, and I would get frustrated to the point of giving up (or maybe that should read "giving in") and retreating to my couch, my office, or somewhere away from everyone for a bit—or even hours at a time. I'm sure I was not a pleasant person to be around in times like those. However, there were times (though not as many as I would have liked) where I managed to pull things together and go on with my daily routine without looking for a corner to curl up in and hide. I might not have been a basket of sunshine in those times, but at least I was making an attempt to move on—some days more successfully than others. It's a miracle my family and colleagues could manage not to slap me around and try to shake me out of it in times like these. Perhaps they actually wanted to do that at one point or another. Perhaps maybe they should have.

I guess, in the big picture, it is a case of mind over matter. However, maybe that phrase means something different than I originally thought. Instead of applying the usual connotation of that saying and allowing the idea of the power of positive thinking to be glorified as the ultimate goal and eventual overwhelming victor in the process, maybe it should be explained differently. Maybe the guiding thought should be that one needs to keep in *mind* what actually *matters* if they are going to be successful. Someone trying to follow that definition as a guiding principle has room to fail and not feel defeated on a constant basis. I know I needed (and still need) plenty of room to fail. Maybe I even need an addition of more personal acreage or at least a wing with several hundred more square feet in order to demarcate the territory taken up by my failures along the way.

Even when I stand in the middle of that yard, field, meadow, or valley of failures, though, there is always a portion of the property standing as a monument to a day—or maybe even an hour—where I did things right. I got out of bed and went to work after only an hour or two of sleep. I took the next pill even though I was pretty sure the side effects were going to kick in. I managed to get through a day in the classroom where I felt like my body was in total revolt and telling me to stop. I got off the couch and went downstairs to spend time with my family instead of being holed up on my upstairs couch, watching a ball game I did not even care about. Did I do these noble things every day? Not even close. Did I even manage to do this at least once a week? Not likely. But from time to time, by the grace of God and the love and support shown to me by my family and colleagues, I did manage to come through and act the way I wanted to or knew I should.

So if every piece of property has that one spot where everything is just right or where the apple tree grows perfectly every season, then every Parkinson's patient—myself included—has that portion of their experience where life is "as it should be." Notice that I did not use that dreaded N word this time. Normal? Not likely to happen. Perfect? Even less likely to exist. Understanding and acting on what really matters in your life? That's the goal for which we all should strive, and it's okay to fail along the way! It's just part of the journey!

CHAPTER 6

Life Lesson 2—It's All a Matter of Perspective

Imagine you are a student in high school. I know. It's a scary time in all our lives that some of us would rather just forget, but play along for a moment. It's Friday and the day of your big chemistry unit test. You've known about it for two weeks, but you kept telling yourself there's "plenty of time" to prepare for the test later. Now it is "later," and you never made yourself find that preparation time you needed. Now what? You try to slide into the room unnoticed by the teacher so she won't see you in your panicked, unprepared state as the bell rings to begin the session. Your mind is racing. How will you ever maintain that 97 percent average you have worked hard to achieve up to this point? What will your parents say when these grades are posted later in the day? Life is not a happy time in this moment. The teacher slides the paper on the desk in front of you, and your mind draws a blank. This is not going to be good! Later that afternoon, you look online and see that, by the grace of God, you made a 72 percent. Your shoulders slump. Your head drops. You know your folks are looking online as well because you've told them today was the big test day. It's not going to be a pleasant conversation at the dinner table tonight.

Now let's change the angle a bit. You are still a student in high school (no, you haven't escaped yet), and you are still facing the same ugly big chemistry unit test in the same class period as the first student. However, things are slightly different in your world. First, you only remembered that there was a big chemistry test in fourth period because you overheard the smart kids in the hallway working together in a study group. At least that's what you think it was because you've never actually been to one of those in your life. At least now you have been given a thirty-minute warning that the test is coming up. How will you ever prepare to defend and maintain the "amazing" 48.9 percent grade you have managed to record in the class to this point? You decide, as usual, that your best bet is to just "wing it" and let the chips (and the points) fall where they may. You breeze through the test in record time—it doesn't take too long when you guess quickly—and then later on, you check the grade online and see a 72 percent on the grade sheet. You let out a holler and wonder how you ever did so well! It sure beats the 47 percent you made on the last test. Maybe you'll be able to get the car keys this weekend after all. Life is good, and it's tacos for dinner tonight!

How is this possible? Two different students…the same grade for each one…and two totally different responses? Easy. It's all a matter of perspective. One student was living in a world where their academic life was always running smoothly and things were under control for the most part. There might be an occasional slipup or forgetful moment, but expectations were high, and success was not a stranger to you. Of course, that meant a significant amount of stress in life, but you found a way to manage it while still emitting the facade to the outside world that you had it all together and nothing could get to you. That was the problem though. It was only a facade. The stinging reality of the bad test grade brought forth the admission that you did not fully prepare. It's a crushing moment, but you have always recovered from these in the past, and you are sure that you will again. It's just the way things go in your world.

On the other side of the ledger is the student who rejoiced in the same grade of 72 percent. This student was not pressured by past successes. Instead, the bar was set so low that they were not even sure there was a bar there to begin with, or it was set so low that they could simply step right over it with the lights turned off. If ignorance is bliss, this student had it made. Life seemed great even if the grades in all seven classes had scores that looked like lottery number picks instead of superior restaurant ratings. The world might be collapsing all around you, but you didn't really take the time to notice or to care about it. Instead, your focus was on the tacos on the dinner menu that night and the elusive car keys that might now be within your reach. Yes, ignorance is bliss, but the reality around you is trying to wake you up to what's coming down the pike. It's just the way things go in your world!

My Parkinson's experience was following the same trajectory of this high school story for years. The problem was, I did not know it. Maybe I did not want to know it, but it was still moving down a similar path whether I liked it or not. From the moment of my diagnosis; through all the initial treatments, record keeping, and questions; to the implementation of medicines that had to be altered, reexamined, and adjusted, I kept trying to tell myself that this was just a bump in the road. Unfortunately, I was not listening to myself very well most days. Instead of remaining positive and shaking off the diagnosis and the treatments as just a temporary issue like the 72 percent on the test, I chose a different path. That road kept me in the same initial stage of reaction and shock the first student experienced. My shoulders stayed slumped. My head remained dropped. I knew people were looking at me and probably wondering what was going on, but I did not accept that as reality. The truth was that I was "losing" the battle against myself, and I didn't even want to accept that fact. Maybe I was happy with the losses? Maybe I didn't think there was anything I could do about it? Maybe it would all just go away? This section of my story will recount some of the stories present as the "losses" began piling up. If only I had known that it's all a matter of perspective!

*****

While I received my official diagnosis of Parkinson's disease in October 2016, in some ways it wasn't until four years later in October 2020 that my treatment actually began. This sounds strange (even to me) when I think about it, but it could be the most accurate description of my journey down the Parkinson's path. Of course, the accuracy of this description did not reveal itself to me immediately. Only after doing some comparisons of my experiences before that date and after that date did things begin to become a bit clearer.

From the time I got home from the doctor's office on the day of my diagnosis, I started trying to formulate a plan of action. Of course, that was more difficult because my head was still spinning trying to figure out the reality of what had just happened in the examination room. My wife and I had a lengthy discussion in an attempt to get on the same page while trying to answer the question that had become the elephant in the room, What next? Looking back on it now, I can see this was the starting point of the diversion of perspectives on my condition.

While shocked about the diagnosis and still a bit uncertain of what it all meant, I went into what I thought was problem-solving mode. Whenever I enter this mode, I feel better about whatever challenge I am facing. If it's a 5K racecourse ahead, I'll find course maps and elevation charts and figure out a strategy for the race. When can I push the pace? Where are the hills? What kind of results have I had in past races on this course or ones that are similar? It feels good to be in this mode because I feel I have a sense of control over my circumstances. That control might not actually exist, but at least I perceive it is there. Either way, my problem-solving mode keeps me feeling busy. The distraction that comes with that sense of "busyness" is comforting because I feel like I am actually accomplishing something. In reality, though, it is a useless exercise in spinning my wheels and not recognizing the changes in my environment. In the example of preparing for a race, even if I know the course well and prepare for a proper pace, I still have to physically run the course according to the plan. Not being able to do that voids any plan you might have formulated beforehand. In the eyes of a professional boxer, the best-conceived plan for your next fight goes right out the window the first time you get punched in the face.

My problem-solving approach led me to start making a to-do list in order to accommodate the doctor's diagnosis and the homework he had assigned me. First, there would need to be a tally sheet, a spreadsheet, or some kind of Google form developed on which I could accurately record the occurrence of my tremors. That was simple enough to manage. I needed more though. One item does not make a good to-do list. Still in problem-solving mode, I quickly devised a plan for tracking my sleep on a spreadsheet as well. Job number 2 on the list? Check!

Over the next two or three days, I came up with many variations of these plans. Some were simple tweaks to the original. Others were complete overhauls that did not last very long in the planning stages. To me, though, what eventually happened to the plans did not matter. The constructive process occupying my mind is what mattered the most. The busier and more "engaged" I was in the planning, the more control and progress I thought would appear. Instead, what I was actually doing was increasing the divide between me and my immediate circle of friends and family. I might have noticed at the time, but I was way too busy! The mistake was thinking my perspective was the only one that mattered. I was wrong…really wrong!

While I was not aware of it at the time, another perspective of my diagnosis was quickly taking shape. Looking back at this early stage in my journey, I wish more than anything I had noticed it. If I had, I could have given it the value it deserved instead of haphazardly ignoring it while in my own little shell of problem-solving. My wife is one of the most practical and straight-to-the-point people I know. Our conversation on the way home from the diagnosis continued once we got home. We covered a lot of ground in this discussion. Who do we tell? How do we break the news? What about our girls? What about work? All these were valid questions, and that might have been part of the problem. As we worked our way through our reactions to the diagnosis and our own ideas of what to do next, I thought more progress was being made than what was actually taking place. Of course, I did not realize this at the time, but I can see now, with the benefit of time and distance, that I was hearing my wife and her ideas, but not really listening to or assigning value to them as I should. I was so concerned about my own thoughts and issues that I was selfishly trying to experience Parkinson's by myself.

This is the weird part. As I look back on these early days from this five-year milestone, I would tell you that if anyone asked me back then how things were going, I would tell them that I felt like I was making progress and that I was lucky to have the most supportive people around me that anyone could ever want. I'm not saying this wasn't the case. In fact, my wife, my kids, and our friends and colleagues were very supportive and wanted to help. The issue, though, was that I was inwardly welcoming them and assuming that was enough while outwardly I was not validating their care, concern, and support. Instead, I was doing quite the opposite. I was retreating from them in order to create what I see now as an intended safe space where I was alone with my thoughts and could try to do my own thing.

In other words, I wanted their help, their concern, and their support, but I did not show them that I valued or appreciated their help, concern, and support. I was king of my own Parkinson's castle, but I was not allowing any loyal subjects to cross the drawbridge. Rather, I let them try to storm the walls, fall helplessly into the moat, and be eaten by the alligators. Some king! Ignoring the subjects and ruling over an empty kingdom! If only I had seen it then. The gates could have been opened, the trumpets could have been sounded, and a grand celebration could have been had by all. Too bad! Instead of playing the role of a grateful and wise king, I was the court jester!

*****

Earlier, I mentioned the possibility that while I was officially diagnosed with Parkinson's in October of 2016, my treatment might not have really begun until October of 2020. Let me explain. In the initial stages, after the tremor logs had been collected and analyzed, the data reviewed and digested, and the prescriptions assigned and filled, it seemed like a regular doctor-patient routine. Something was ailing me. I was sent to a doctor. An examination was performed. Medicine was issued. Life went on. For a while, that seemed correct and appropriate. There were struggles with the medication that led to nausea. There were adjustments made. New medicines were prescribed and taken. It was all a vicious cycle, but in the moment, all seemed well. Once again, though, that was my perspective—one that was tainted by my desire not to cause any commotion, keep my head down, do what I was told by the medical professionals, and not question the results or the process.

As in other phases of my life, Parkinson's was taking control of my thought process. I continued thinking that as long as I was busy and thought I was doing the right thing that it would all be okay. Maybe that was denial. Looking back at it now, I'm sure it was. I was "happiest" when I could be by myself, not have to interact, and keep things in what I was certain was a safe and secure personal bubble. My efforts to remain safe and secure in my own space, though, were driving a wedge between me and those who cared about me and for me. People like my wife, my daughters, and my colleagues thought they were, in some respects, losing me. As was also usually the case in these early stages, I had no idea that I was the one causing this sense of loss.

My medications and their overall effectiveness were always a point of contention in the first few years of my treatment. Most days, I would answer people who asked me how the treatments were going with the traditional response of "As expected" or "Things seem to be going well." I truly believed those responses were true and also served the purpose of being what I was "supposed to say" when asked that question. Nobody would want to hear the medications were totally ineffective and not having any impact on my condition. Even if that were the case, why would I tell someone that? Why indeed? In the moment, I wanted to believe so badly that the doctors were right on top of things and that they knew exactly what to prescribe and there would be no reason to experience a trial of one drug or dosage in order to see if it worked or not. Surely, I believed, all those issues had been worked out on other patients, and I would be the beneficiary of their experiences. My treatment was supposed to go on without a hitch. Nothing was supposed to be questioned, challenged, or reevaluated. All those beliefs grew inside my head each and every day. It is said that if you hear a lie long enough that you will start to believe it represents truth. That was me—telling myself the lies I wanted to hear and saying them so loudly they drowned out the chorus of the reality that was chanting in the same arena in which I existed.

Husbands should always listen to their wives. This is especially true during difficult circumstances. As the initial stages of my treatment and prescriptions wore on and weeks became months, my wife was having a difficult time figuring me out. Of course, at the time this was happening, I was blind to it all because I was still living the dream in "The meds are working and it's going to be fine" stage of life. Days would come along where my wife might offer a glimmer of hope to my style of existence by acknowledging that I was indeed having a "good day" with my tremors or other symptoms. I would find out much later, though, that those were just an attempt not to face her perspective that I was changing so quickly in front of her that she was not sure how to recapture me and bring me back to my usual self. I wish now that I had known what I was doing to my family. I wish I could have seen the reality of the situation and appreciated their perspectives more than what I did at the time, which was to not even acknowledge them at all.

All of 2017 and most of 2018 continued in this same pattern. I was taking my meds, following the rules, trying to manage the symptoms at work while teaching, and playing the role of the dutiful graduate school student closing in on his doctoral degree. It was the latter of those roles that provided an opportunity for me to get a better view of the reality of my existence as it was seen by others. In December of 2018, I was graduating from Piedmont College with my doctorate, and graduation day had arrived. The ceremony was one of the most exciting days of my life as I was hooded, walked across the stage to get my diploma, and then attended a wonderful luncheon with all the doctoral graduates. It was truly a day to remember. My family was all there, some of my colleagues made the trip to take part in the ceremonies, and tons of pictures were taken to commemorate the event. The pictures actually did more than simply serve as a keepsake. They gave me a chance to see myself as others had been seeing me for months.

After the graduation luncheon, I viewed most of the photos that had been posted on Facebook. I was looking forward to seeing the pictures and reading the comments, but the pictures grabbed my attention the most.

"Who is that old guy wearing the robes?"

These were the first words that came to mind when I saw the photo of me walking down the aisle toward the stage to get hooded.

"That can't be me!"

The truth is, however, that it *was* me, and I did not like what I was seeing. The frailness and the overall "old man" image I saw staring back at me in the photos was jarring.

"Is this really the way I look?"

It was at this point I began to ask some important questions of myself. I wanted to figure out how I had gotten to this point. More importantly, I wanted to figure out what to do going forward so I could change this appearance. I think, though, it involved more than just changing the external. The internal needed some work as well. I guess there's always a catch! Physical changes can be mapped out, scheduled, placed into a routine. You eat well, work out, and get enough rest, and the external portion usually comes out well. It's not as easy or straightforward to change the internal. That requires more work, more discipline, and more support. At least going forward, I would know I had the support. The question remained if I had the mental discipline to "put in the time" and work at it.

The new year started in January 2019 with high hopes. It was kind of like making New Year's resolutions for my Parkinson's life. Instead of the traditional resolutions of saving more money, losing some weight, trying to stop some annoying bad habits, or something else of that kind, I wanted to recapture my old self. Maybe *old* was not the best choice of word to describe my goal. Let's say "previous" self instead of "old." I did not want to be associated with anything old at that point.

For the first few months, like any traditional New Year's resolutions, I did pretty well. I tried to remain more positive. I tried to spend more time around the family. I tried to keep my spirits up at work and not be one to complain about everything. Most people don't realize how difficult it is for teachers not to complain about so many things. It's what we do! There would be no need for a teacher's lounge if there weren't grievances to be aired and problems to complain about. It just wouldn't be the same. However, I digress.

I made it through the doldrums of winter and entered the spring season on an upward climb. Then life got busy, and I started to backslide. It did not take long before I was back in the negative routine of isolating myself whenever possible, trying to ignore any meaningful conversations about my condition, and not really caring what anyone else thought. I was back on track to releasing the "old man" in me again, and it was frustrating. The fact that I recognized what was happening was a step in the right direction though. It bought me a little more time trying to fight off the regression, but by the end of the school year and the start of my summer break, it was too late. My old self had returned. The only difference this time was, I was less certain that I was doing the right thing with my current medications. It was beginning to dawn on me that what my wife had been trying to tell me all along was true. The medications, the patches, and all the treatments were not having any effect.

Maybe the summer break would be just what I needed. Instead of viewing it as a time to get a break from the classroom routines, the supervision duties, and the lesson plans that make up a teacher's world for nine months of the year, I needed to get a break from my personal stresses and find some way to rekindle the drive I had in the early stages of the year when the resolutions were new and the body didn't feel so old. No such luck though. I tried getting more involved with my golf game but wasn't playing well. That, in and of itself, was not the frustrating part. I was starting to feel more and more restricted in my movements and swinging of the clubs. I wondered for the first time if my days on the golf course were numbered. There I was…thinking like an old man again!

I kept wearing the medical patch and taking the other medications that made up my pharmaceutical routine. Soon, summer was over, and the school bells would be ringing. They would probably match the ringing in my head with all my frustrating thoughts bouncing off one lobe of my brain and onto another. Nothing seemed clear. Nothing seemed right. I was withdrawing from the world. What made it different this time around was that I knew what

I was doing! There was none of the usual positivity centered around the falsehoods of thinking the meds were doing their job. There was no satisfaction in trying to play the role of the dutiful patient anymore. There were questions upon questions and no answers anywhere around. I was getting to a breaking point. What I did not realize, though, was exactly how close I was to that point!

*****

To be honest, the fall 2019 semester was kind of a blur. Days and weeks ran together too easily. The hectic school-teacher routine seemed to have me running on the gerbil wheel faster than ever before, with only momentary pauses for a sip from the suspended water bottle that was my home life. The faster I would run to try and keep up with things at work, the more exhausted I would get. It's no wonder I was so tired. The gerbil wheel doesn't exactly give you a great measure of progress. It only reacts to your expenditure of effort. I wish I had figured that out sooner. I'd have slowed down some and not worn out the gears on about three of those wheels in the four months leading up to December 2019!

Those four months led me to the breaking point. My "routine" had become well established. The alarm clock would go off at five o'clock on weekday mornings. The next few minutes were dedicated to an interpersonal debate whether or not I really wanted to go to work. Some mornings, the "old man" won out in the battle of rationalizations.

"The tremors were too tough last night. I just can't do this today!"

Other mornings, the more professional side would win.

"There's too much to do today at school. I can't afford to miss another day!"

There I was. It's 5:10 a.m., and already the gerbil wheel was spinning at full force. I haven't even gotten out of bed yet, and I'm already tired of running. By 5:45 a.m., I'm in the car and off to another day at the races. How many revolutions would I make on the wheel today? Would anyone else notice my futile efforts to create a scenario in which I could just be a regular teacher for the day? How soon would that three-ten bell ring so that I could get back in my car, drive the twenty-five miles home, and retreat for the rest of the evening into a personal shell? This was the way my world worked. Instead of being a teacher who just happened to have Parkinson's, I had become a full-time Parkinson's patient who tried to act like a teacher nine months out of the year. Not only was my "old man" self winning; he had run through the end zone, spiked the football in my face, gone to the sidelines to claim the trophy, and trampled on me on the way back to the locker room celebration.

It was decision time for me as the Christmas break started. I was tired of the running. I was tired of not feeling like I was making any progress. I was done with the tremors causing countless nights of restlessness. I wanted to change. I wanted to be "normal" again. Yes, I said it. I wanted to be "normal." I guess I should have been more careful what I wished for. My "breaking point" moment involved the rationalization that if the medical patches and the pills were not working, then why even use them or take them? I had tried this a few weeks prior to this breaking point and thought I had gathered some important data to support my move toward normalcy. I stopped wearing the patch for about four or five days. To me, those days seemed just like the countless days of wearing the patch. My scientific brain needed some more confirmation, so I went back to the patch the next day. I was so nauseous and out of it that day (not to mention it was a day filled with tremors) that I felt the experiment was complete. No more medications for this old man! I was done! My New Year's resolution for 2020—back to the normal world of no medications. Surely that would be the answer! I had even "tested" it out to make sure it made sense. Of course, how much can one learn during a one-day experiment on anything? No matter! I was ready to face the world unmedicated. I was ready to try to be me again.

As you have probably figured out by this point, my decision ranks among some of the worst choices in my life. Change that! It was probably the worst decision in my life. You would think that a logical person like me would have been able to see this coming. I would like to have thought so as well, but that would have required me to be in a rational and logical place at that very moment. Breaking points, by their very definition, are not laced with logic and sound reasoning skills. That's why people break under them. Stupid choices are at the top of the menu for diners in the café of a crisis. In fact, they are the appetizer, the main course, and you get a double helping of them for dessert! It might be delicious in the moment, but you most certainly pay for it in the long term.

January and February were two of the longest months I can remember in this Parkinson's journey. There I was, trying to run the gerbil wheel at full speed with no fuel to maintain my conditioning. Even the respite of being at home didn't provide the break I needed in order to get off the wheel. Some days, the wheel spun even faster at home. When I would try to find my protected space and comfortable shell of retreat, my brain would still be in high gear.

"What am I going to do about these tremors? Shouldn't they be going away? What now?"

As crazy and misguided as these self-questioning sessions seem now, at the time they seemed proper and more productive than destructive. I was so convinced to be successful and normal without medication that I did not want to even come close to admitting I had made a bad choice. I had rationalized my condition so much that it seemed logical to think that the symptoms should disappear with no medications working against them. I had tried the prescribed pills, and those didn't seem to work, so surely taking nothing would be the answer. Sometimes I wonder how I ever made it to March!

The other downside to my January and February 2020 existence was my self-consciousness of how I presented myself to others, especially at work. My students all knew about my condition. There had been prayers and wonderfully supportive comments from many of them along the way. Deep down inside, I knew they cared and wanted me to be well. However, the not-so-logical side of me was entirely convinced. I did not want to be the "Parkinson's teacher," the guy with the shaky left hand and bouncing left foot that was kind of a distraction in the classroom. I just wanted to be an English teacher, a coach, and a mentor to these kids. In my nonmedicated state, I thought I should be able to conquer all these obstacles easily. It's a shame how much energy I wasted trying to do then what was truly an impossible task. It would have been so much easier to sit back and just accept my condition for what it was and just do my job. Of course, that would have been easier, but I was not in a frame of mind to do what was easy. I wanted to do things my way because certainly I knew what was best for me. Wrong again!

*****

It was March 13, 2020, when the world changed. In a way, it was fitting that this fell on a Friday the 13th as it was a scary time for all of us. Educators like me had been keeping close tabs on this mysterious story about some illness called COVID-19. We did not really know what was going to happen, but we all felt pretty certain it was not going to be a pretty sight. I had just finished up broadcasting a high school baseball game on our campus and was packing up the car to head home. Neurologically speaking, it had been a pretty good day. The tremors were mostly in check, there had been no serious bouts with nausea, and I felt pretty strong. The Spartans baseball team had just won their game in a convincing fashion, and the parents working the concession stand had even brought me my favorite broadcaster's dinner—a hot dog and a Diet Coke! Please, no lectures on the lack of nutritional value of this meal. It was delicious!

As I got in my car, my phone started blowing up with text messages. Our school was going to go "virtual" starting on the upcoming Monday. I had thought this might be a possibility, but the reality of the text message was a bit jarring. Instead of driving in to work every day, I would be in my home office teaching the kids through Zoom classes and video lessons. While my "teacher brain" was trying to figure out the logistics of working from home, the Parkinson's patient in me was experiencing mixed feelings. Teaching from home would reduce the possibility of being "noticed" so much for my tremors. There would even be some days where I would not need to have my camera on the entire time during a class period. This seemed like a step in the right direction. I could just be a teacher. This was what I had wanted for so long. I had no idea that idea was so far-fetched that it would take a global pandemic to make it a reality. In this new virtual setup, my personal gerbil wheel would be slowed down remarkably. I could even enjoy the water breaks now more than ever.

The initial stages of virtual learning were challenging, but I soon embraced the concept wholeheartedly. I could sleep a little later, enjoy my morning coffee at a leisurely pace, wear shorts or sweats instead of khakis or slacks, and focus on the lessons and assisting my students more individually than I had for quite some time in the in-person instructional model. Life was good. As it turned out, though, it was too good to be true. Like those amazing doodads on late-night infomercials that would change your world for only $19.99, this virtual learning setup was going to turn out to be too good to be true for the Parkinson's patient in me.

When it became evident that the remainder of the school year would be virtual, I was excited and somewhat relieved. What I wasn't expecting, though, was that the comforts of teaching from home that I enjoyed so much were actually making me too comfortable. My routine had changed. There were no more 5:00 a.m. wakeup calls; no frantic interstate driving to get to work; no ball games, practices, or help sessions to handle after the school hours were done. It was just my students and me—connected through Zoom—and I did not have to go anywhere! It was an introvert's paradise! That was the problem. Since I did not have to venture out into the real world due to the stay-at-home orders in our state and the other COVID-19 restrictions put into place, my comfortable shell of home I was so used to retreating into at the end of my time rushing through my day had now become my entire day. There were no worries about if the medications were working or not. It did not matter. Nobody would be able to tell if I was having a bad Parkinson's day or not. My "fortress of solitude" had become so invincible that I was really hoping to never have to leave it again. If I was going to stay in my shell for so long, who needs medication? What had started as a global emergency and briefly transformed into a professional adjustment was now more serious than ever before. It was the crutch I was using to embolden my decision to stop taking my medication. That was all I needed at that point...another excuse!

This is one point in my Parkinson's journey where my perspective and that of my wife were perfectly aligned, at least in the moment. While she was adjusting her schedule for her students (she's an elementary teacher) to meet the virtual requirements, she was pleased I did not have to travel to work each day and that my crazy afternoon schedules had been pretty much reduced to nothing. Just a few weeks before the start of the pandemic, we had discussed ways to slow down my crazy gerbil-like schedule. I had even gone as far as to create a calendar for the refrigerator with all my practices, tournaments, broadcasting obligations, and all-important date nights listed for the months of March, April, and May. In hindsight, maybe I should have seen the need to slow down a bit earlier. In the moment, though, I felt I was supposed to be able to do it all—with or without medication. The stress and the busyness made me crazy, but in a strange kind of way, I embraced the "crazy" and struggled through it. At least it gave me something to complain about. Those complaints, though, when directed toward my wife, always met the same retort: "You chose this, so you can't complain about it." Once again, she was right!

*****

Having made it through the end of the school year, I had been hoping for society to return to its prepandemic state. If that happened, I would be able to get outside during the summer break and work on my failing golf game and get a little vitamin D from the sun. Of course, that did not happen. May, June, and July were much like the previous three months. The lockdowns continued, restrictions grew a bit more stringent, and my hermit-like existence received another boost. Even if I thought I might like to get outside, I was very comfortable where I was. There was the challenge of trying to find sports to watch on TV since most of the leagues had been shut down due to the pandemic, but I managed just as well. If there was a fringe sport I had heard about, ESPN was trying to fill programming slots with it, and that was okay by me.

While my appreciation for German soccer grew during this downtime, another new facet of my Parkinson's journey began to develop. In mid to late June, I started having what could best be described as gagging attacks. I would feel overwhelmingly nauseous and would start coughing and gagging. It was like the worst dry heaving experience I had ever encountered. Not pleasant! These attacks started sporadically. I would have two or three a week. Soon, they became more constant as the summer break wound down. By early August, during my preparation to return to school, the attacks were coming on almost on a daily basis. I tried various techniques to combat these attacks, but nothing seemed to have an effect on them. It never even dawned on me that the lack of medication might be playing some role in all this.

The first week of August rolled around, and it was back to the campus to teach in a hybrid setup. Students could choose to come to school in person or join the classes virtually. It took some getting used to, but it seemed to be a good option as the pandemic was still surging in our area as school started back. What was also surging was the declining state of my health. The bills for choosing to go off my medication back in December were now coming due, and it was worse than getting any credit card statement in the mail that I can remember.

Throughout August and September, I probably missed more days of work than I was actually present for. On multiple occasions, I became ill at work with the gagging attacks and was sent home by the nurse. They still could not take any chances with COVID-19 still hanging around. On certain days, my blood pressure would skyrocket and cause dizzy spells and nausea. This, of course, created challenging days at work. One September morning I was so nauseous and hit with elevated blood pressure that I went to the emergency room for treatment. It wasn't a very productive trip as I did not get many answers other than to check with the local GI doctor as well as my neurologist, Dr. Raju. I kind of knew that was coming somewhere down the line during all these struggles. Perhaps the logical side of my brain should have forced its way through a bit sooner and convinced me that visiting the neurologist might be a good idea.

My GI doctor recommended an endoscopy procedure that would check not only the lining of my esophagus but also the upper ends of my bowels for any issues that might be causing these attacks. During that procedure, they would also stretch my throat slightly to prevent any swallowing issues that might arise from these gagging attacks. In my discussions with Dr. Raju, he agreed that the endoscopy was a good idea, but he was also able to shed a little more light on potential causes of the attacks.

"Do you consider yourself to be working in a high-stress environment?" he asked.

It was all I could do not to laugh. "High stress" was putting it mildly. I'm a teacher surrounded by tenth graders all day. Of course, it's high stress!

The discussion then took a turn that I had been wanting to avoid but was pretty certain was coming sometime soon. Dr. Raju asked the question I did not want to answer.

"How is the medicine treating you?"

There it was, the question I could no longer avoid. It was time to see what happened next. I told Dr. Raju that I had been totally off any Parkinson's medications for the last nine months. There, I said it! Dr. Raju paused for a moment and then responded with an answer that I did not expect.

"You're doing better than expected for someone totally off the medications for that long."

If only he had stopped there, I could have made a justifiable defense of my actions. But of course, there was more.

"However, you can't expect to control your tremors with no medicine at all. We will need to find the right formula for your case."

I knew it! There's always a "however" in there somewhere when I think things are about to go my way lately or prove me right in my decisions. While part of me was displeased that I did not get to proclaim "I told you so" to the world, another part of me was relieved and excited that maybe this was the moment when I could finally get some real answers.

As the discussion continued, a remarkable revelation regarding my wife and my differing perspectives on my Parkinson's journey came to light. Dr. Raju asked me if I had experienced any bouts of depression. When I heard that, I wanted to laugh again. Depression? I'm not depressed. I'm gagging my guts out. My wife, though, beat me to the punch and told Dr. Raju that she was almost certain I was depressed. I can only imagine the quizzical look I must have given her in that moment. She told Dr. Raju about my life since the school went virtual in March and how I had confined myself so much to my at-home existence that instead of using the time of seclusion to spend more quality time with my family, I was doing just the opposite. I was drifting further and further away. She and the girls were losing me again!

I guess those who are experiencing depression are the last to realize it is happening. However, this is yet another instance where I discovered the difference in perspectives that were held about my Parkinson's experience. I was so caught up in figuring out how to adjust to the changing environment with my job that I did not focus on the amazing opportunity that had been thrust upon me with the stay-at-home orders and ability to work from home. Maybe that was God's way of telling me to back things down a bit in my life and appreciate what I had that was really important to me. It's a shame I did not see it soon enough to take full advantage of the situation. Instead, it took a stunning revelation from my wife in a doctor's office to snap me back to attention that something serious was indeed going on here. It's no wonder I love her so much!

It was at this critical point on my Parkinson's timeline where events took a turn for the better. Finally, a plan was being put into place that would hopefully bring an end to the horrible gagging attacks and also get me back to a more manageable state of mind. I had been through so much in the past nine months that I was ready for a change.

The new plan involved a two-prong attack on my issues. First, in response to the tremors and lack of mobility that I had been experiencing, Dr. Raju increased my Sinemet (carbidopa-levodopa pill) dosage by a factor of three. Doing this would be the most effective way to get the needed dopamine into my system. While the higher dosage of dopamine did have an increased risk of nausea (of course it does), the increased combination of the two medicines should be enough to combat the issue if I could get through a week or two of the dosage and get used to having it in my system. In order to survive that period as well as any future nausea issues, he prescribed Zofran (soon to be my new best friend for a few weeks) to fight off the nausea and even help with the gagging sensations.

While not exactly thrilled with the prospect of more nauseated days, I had learned my lesson. Don't stop taking your medications! My wife would make sure this mantra was indelibly engraved on my soul from this day forward…just in case I got any wild ideas on my own in the future. Dr. Raju also had a plan for the gagging attacks and the depression. He prescribed an antidepressant (citalopram) that would improve my mood after only about a week or two of the prescription. It would also serve as a medication to distract my Parkinson's from attacking the nerves that can control or regulate esophageal spasms. This, he believed, could have been the cause of the gagging attacks, along with the issues found by my GI doctor. This sounded like great news to me. A better mood, more mobility, and reduced gagging attacks? I'm in, even if I have to get through some more bouts of nausea to get there! As it stands now, Dr. Raju was correct, and this is the medicine regimen I am still on today. Has it worked? Just ask my wife and kids! I've been more involved at home, watched more family movies together than in past months, have been noticeably more mobile at work, and can even swing the golf clubs a bit more freely. I don't think Tiger Woods has anything to worry about regarding competition from me. I still play bad golf, but I can at least enjoy it more at this point.

So where does all this leave me? Am I the high school student who meant to study, never found time to do so, and stresses out when the test comes, or am I the student who is so oblivious to his surroundings that he's not even aware a test is coming and is just happy to survive? I think I'm a little bit of both. Some days I know are going to be challenging, but I still don't do everything right to prepare. On those days, survival is the goal, and I truly am delighted just to make it to the end of the day in one piece. At other times, I try hard not to worry about the circumstances of my Parkinson's experience to a great extent and try to coast through the day in as carefree a manner as possible. Sure, I'll still have failures on those days, but maybe they won't bother me as much as on other days. What I really wish, though, is to be the third kind of student: the one who knows the test is coming, diligently prepares and motivates themselves to do well, aces the test all the time, and then walks confidently down the hallway to meet the test coming up in the next class period. That would be nice, but I'm not quite there yet, and I don't know if I ever will get there. I guess it's just a matter of perspective!

CHAPTER 7

Life Lesson 3—the Pillars of the Parkinson's Pathway

That early October day in 2016 when the diagnosis of my Parkinson's condition was revealed, I remember experiencing a variety of emotions. Of course, I was shaken a bit by the news and was caught between trying to physically comprehend what had just happened and emotionally trying to prepare for what came next. I was also quite fearful. There were a lot of unknowns in this diagnosis. Even the doctor told me my progression could follow a variety of paths.

One possibility was that I would maintain a slow and steady progression of deterioration until I reached a point where I would need complete assistance with my quality of daily life. Another possibility was remaining exactly as I was at the point of diagnosis for what could be a myriad of years. Any length of time from three years all the way to twenty-five years of stagnation (a good thing in the progression of the disease) was possible for some patients, especially those who are diagnosed at the early onset stage of life. In a weird way, I was also experiencing a bit of relief upon hearing the news. At least at this point, I had an answer. There was no more mystery as to what the medical issues could be. In an odd twist, it was better in my mind to know that the answer could be devastating in the long term than to not know anything at all.

Finally, I found myself feeling very curious. I wanted to know more about the journey through Parkinson's others had taken. By gaining more information and anecdotes from people who have been down this very path, maybe I could feel a bit more comfortable in my own journey's steps. That is the goal for me in this life lesson section of my story. Hopefully, my discovery of the four "pillars" along the Parkinson's pathway described in this section will assist someone else who is on the same road and fighting the same battles. We can all grow together!

*****

Any good engineer or architect knows for a structure to be sound and safe, there needs to be a strong and properly constructed foundation. It would do no good to have the world's best design for a skyscraper or new corporate building and then build that structure on the wrong kind of soil or base it on an improper foundation. In many respects, constructing my journey down my "pathway" that is life with Parkinson's involves the same sentiment. If I have all the book knowledge regarding Parkinson's stored in my brain but then I fail to "ground" myself properly, the structure is destined to fail. For my purposes, I imagine my life and journey through Parkinson's as a squared-off structure with solid boundaries and four pillars of support, one at each corner, providing the stability needed to maintain the integrity of the structure. For me, the size of the pillars can vary based on how much of a load is placed on or near that corner or section of my life structure. Additional "stories" or layers to my life structure would require more strength on the part of the pillars. If an area or section of my life structure is damaged or weakened, that corner support pillar is not carrying as heavy a load but is ready to fully support that section when the crisis has been resolved and the reconstruction has been completed.

That last point is one that needs to be emphasized. While I feel I have discovered my four pillars to support my life structure, just having the pillars is not enough unless I build upon them and give them something to support. Inactivity on my part results in my pillars not being utilized to their full extent. Why would you build a support system when there is no structure to support? Additionally, it is important to recognize that damage or weakness will happen along the pathway. A structure's reception of damage or weakness is not the responsibility of the pillars of support. Instead, it must be accepted as truth that bad things will happen along the journey, and when they do, the pillars of support will be needed to provide strength and secure footing for the damage to be repaired. For example, just because I have found the pillars I need in my journey does not mean that on the days when my tremors are out of control or my days get flipped so that I think noon is midnight and vice versa that it is because I do not have strong support in that portion of my life structure. It means that when the tough times come (and they will), the structure can be rebuilt with the support of the pillar there as a framework and guide to completing the reconstruction.

Discovering my four pillars of support was not a complicated task, but it was one that was rather time-consuming. While I was eager to continue living in the most usual way possible, I recognized early on in my journey that I would need some help. It sounds reasonable, but it was a challenge for me because it would require me to admit that I was not in total control of my situation and that I needed someone else. After much deliberation, consternation, frustration, and perspiration, my four pillars rose from the ground and began to form the foundation for my journey through Parkinson's: friends, formula, flexibility, and finish.

Pillar Number 1—Friends

I'll be honest. In mapping out this section, I could not get the lyrics to the theme song from the TV series *Friends* out of my head. Now you probably will have the same issue since I mentioned it. But think about it. It works.

"So no one told you life was gonna be this way…"

How true this is for a Parkinson's patient! I know that was the case in my life. Even after injuring my shoulder and setting the fateful diagnosis plan in motion, I was not even thinking about something as serious as Parkinson's. Maybe it was a pinched nerve, but not a life-altering disease. The denial I experienced at the moment of diagnosis struck me as hard as a rake handle smacking me in the face after I stepped on the tongs at the other end. It requires acceptance. I got smacked in the face with the rake handle because it was a natural reaction to the controlling circumstances. I did not want it to happen, but it did, and now I had to deal with it. I could stand there cursing the rake for hitting me in the face, or I could manage the pain I was feeling in the moment by asking for help in the form of an ice pack or bandage from someone nearby. Too many times, I chose standing and cursing the rake inexplicably, knowing that wasn't going to change anything. My use of colorful metaphors was not going to make the bruise on my face go away. However, asking for and getting help from a friend with an ice pack would help me control the immediate circumstances while also allow me to begin to move on from the situation.

Early on in my journey, there were many people standing close by with symbolic ice packs ready to offer assistance. My graduate school cohort members such as Dr. David Sells, Dr. Nancy Kluge, and others were there to help me refocus my life on my graduate school work while offering words of encouragement and, in David's case, some very entertaining matches and/or distractions on the golf course as we played many "friendly" rounds along the way. At work, friends and colleagues such as Lauri Fields, Jami and Brad Denton, Tammy Hughes, Tami Miller, Jennifer Thomas, Jeremy Beauchamp, Ellie Kenworthy, and others I'm sure I am forgetting were there all along the way to offer a kind word, cover a class (or two or ten) if needed, make me laugh when I needed it most, or just be there to listen when I would get into a low spot or stumble along my pathway. There were days, I am sure, when they were probably tired of me griping, complaining, and struggling to do even the most mundane parts of my work as a teacher, but they still managed to be there and just listened to all my rantings and ravings when my world would get crazy.

This first pillar calls for action. Those of us on the Parkinson's pathway may not always cry out with a loud voice in need of support in all circumstances. Some, like myself in the early stages of my journey, are content and convinced we can handle the situation by ourselves. We do not want to burden the world around us with our problems when there are so many other important things going on that need attention. My advice to fellow Parkinson's patients is, find that one person with whom you can be vulnerable. Find that one person who you know will make you laugh or listen to you cry if needed. Every Parkinson's patient wants and needs support from a closely knit group of friends. Sometimes, though, we have a tough time getting that message across.

"It's like you're always stuck in second gear, when it hasn't been your day, your week, your month or even your year…"

I can relate to this one all too well! I might have found myself stuck in every gear on the stick and not just second gear along this journey. I think the portion of my journey down the pathway that presented the need for the discovery of this initial pillar was my early frustration with the medications I had been prescribed. I do not consider myself a great medical patient, but I do firmly believe I am a good rule follower. If the doctor tells me I need to take x number of pills x times each day in order to get the desired result or to feel better, I tend to believe the doctor, and I try to do my best to follow the instructions to the letter. Notice I said "try." I might consider myself to be a good rule follower, but that doesn't always make it true in other people's perspectives.

In my mind, if I have followed the doctor's instructions (or at least most of them most of the time), I should expect to get the desired results. When I was taking the early dosages of my meds and not getting the relief from the tremors I expected, I was not a pleasant person to be around. Grumpy Cat would have nothing on me! In these times, I needed that someone who could set me straight when it was called for, reassure me that all was going to be okay in the big picture, and of course, remind me I needed to be following all the doctor's directions all the time if I wanted to have expectations of results.

A colleague of mine, Tim Ball, and a friend of mine, Mr. Dana Davis, play this role for me and provide the support I need in critical moments. Coach Ball, an anatomy teacher at my school, has a unique way of making me see things in a less serious manner when I get too wound up about things not going well. Not only does Coach Ball "nag" me about my loyalty to the Auburn Tigers but he also has the ability to make me forget about the issue or crisis at hand and just focus on getting through the day—or even just the moment. Coach Ball's scientific background proves helpful when I have questions about the reactions in the body to certain medical interventions, and his neurology knowledge is quite extensive, though he would play it down. There would be mornings at work when I come in frustrated, exhausted, or just unfocused, and I would "just happen" to run into Coach Ball at the coffee station. Within moments, I am laughing or responding to some quip he's made, and I have forgotten about (at least temporarily) whatever the crisis at hand was in that moment. His support and reassurance have gone a long way to providing the support I need to my life structure.

Dana Davis has been a longtime friend of the family. About fifteen years ago, he and his wife came and visited my family while we were spending a year living and teaching in Qingdao, China, through a mission effort sponsored by my school. Dana has endured a number of hardships by battling cancer for years, but his spirit is never beaten down. Showing the godly heart of a servant, Dana always places others before himself and looks to find new ways to serve. Dana's friendship and support has been invaluable to me. While I don't see him on campus as often as I would like, he always stops and checks on me when he has a chance. No question, prayer request, or medical update ever seems too off-the-wall or irrelevant to Dana when we visit, and I will always appreciate his continued support of my journey. I rest easier knowing I have a true prayer warrior on my side. Everyone should be so lucky!

"I'll be there for you [when the rain starts to pour]. I'll be there for you [like I've been there before]. I'll be there for you..."

Parkinson's patients would probably all agree that there are days along the journey where "the rain starts to pour." These are dark and somber times and can occur suddenly and without warning. You can be having a great week physically and be feeling like you can conquer the world in a single stroke, and then it all comes crashing down around you with a sleepless night, an unexpected reaction to medication, some bizarrely vivid dream or nightmare that jolts you awake in a kicking and screaming fit at 2:00 a.m., or just a downtrodden or depressed moment where you wade into the pool of self-pity and doubt. No matter the event that brings about these "downpours" in your Parkinson's life, you always seem to feel like you never saw it coming and there's not an umbrella in sight or within reach.

Many of my "downpour" days are a result of sleep issues I face on a pretty constant basis. Even though I would say my sleep patterns have improved to some degree in the last year, there are still many more instances than I would like where I am awake all night or have incredibly vivid dreams that jolt me awake suddenly and disrupt the sleep patterns. These usually feature me kicking out or punching the air suddenly in response to the action in my dream. Luckily, I have not kicked or punched out in my wife's direction too many times. That would not be good for anyone, especially me! In one of my more recent disruptions, I dreamed as clear as day that a rather tall package had been delivered to my front door. It was not a box but an odd-shaped package wrapped in brown paper. It seemed to be moving and making rather weird noises. I opened the front door to inspect the package, and an ostrich broke free from the packaging and chased me through the entire lower level of my house, biting at me constantly while I was swinging and kicking wildly! No, I did not have the late-night burrito special from the gas station food menu! This was a standard version of one of those things that make me "go bump in the night."

On the days following such sleepless nights, friends and colleagues at work have come to my rescue more than once. Sometimes it might be covering a class for me for a few minutes while I get more coffee or a Diet Coke to combat the exhaustion of the moment. Maybe I needed copies made and my to-do list was not getting done. Colleagues have stepped in and helped me get caught up, even on the craziest of days. I am sincerely blessed to work in a place where there are high levels of concern and compassion for others. It's these kinds of people that I need when my "rain" starts to fall. They've been there before, and I feel certain they will continue to be there for me.

"No one could ever know me. No one could ever see me. Seems you're the only who knows what it's like to be me. Someone to face the day with, make it through all the rest with. Someone I'll always laugh with. Even at my worst, I'm best with you…"

As a Parkinson's patient, there are days when I wish "no one could ever know me" and "no one could ever see me." These feelings surface on days of higher degrees of self-consciousness due to tremors acting up or when I have issues speaking slowly and clearly enough for my students to take notes in class. In these moments, I wish I could just curl up in a little ball somewhere and become invisible. Surely, I think, the students notice what's going on during my rougher days in the classroom. I want to believe they understand. Deep down inside, I know that to be the case, but it does not make the apprehension any less disconcerting. These desires to be unknowable and invisible are most likely what aided my movement toward depression within the past twelve months. Since I have been on the antidepression medicine, I have noticed a stronger sense of confidence in the classroom and less apprehension on days when my mobility is not up to par.

In some ways, my students have become more than just students in my classes. They have become friends who lend support in times of need, in their own unique and teenaged ways. It might sound weird for a teacher to think of students as friends. There's a matter of professional distance that needs to be maintained for a classroom to function well. However, I offer evidence to the contrary. Sometimes, the lesson on the board at the front of the classroom is not the most important material of the day. Sometimes, there's a need for a life lesson, and the students find ways to pass that assignment with flying colors.

In the 2019–2020 school year, I was blessed with an amazing class of students for my English 12 class. Many of the students had been in my English 10 and/or English 11 classes, so there was a sense of connection already developed. These students had seen the earlier stages of my battle with Parkinson's, and many of them had written notes or emails to me offering encouragement and support. Out of all these students, though, I had a couple that came to be known as my watchdogs. They could tell when I was having a rough day and almost always made it a point to talk to me before class or afterward and just check in to make sure I was doing okay that day. It doesn't sound like much, but it meant a great deal to me on the days when the struggles were real. A couple of times, they even told me they had been praying for me and my family. That was incredible! It's nice to know that even on the roughest of days, there are friends like that to "face the day with" and "make it through all the rest with." In short, we should all have friends like these!

Pillar Number 2—Formula

Let's face it. There's a reason I teach English and literature for a living. It's simple… I do not want to teach science or math. To say those subjects are not my strong suit would be a gross under-statement. Even with my father being a biochemist and my younger brother teaching some kind of advanced math at the college level that seems like it might as well be a study in ancient hieroglyphics, that base of knowledge and comprehension did not find their way into my brain on a long-term basis. I knew just enough in those areas to be dangerous and survive high school biology and a couple of required algebra courses. Many people say they are confused with "new math." I barely survived the "old math," and I think I turned out just fine. The science I need I can locate through Siri or Google, and the math I need can be done for me with my online grading program. Problem solved.

While not being an expert scientist or some mathematical prodigy, I do have an appreciation for what lies at the foundation of many of the principles of those fields. Both of those academic areas often require the use of complicated, advanced formulas in order to be successful or discover elusive answers. Without the vital formula fully intact and precisely structured, the chances of reaching the proper solution for a given problem are greatly reduced. Something as simple as a misplaced sign or symbol, an improperly copied number, or a failure to follow a certain sequential order of steps or procedures can lead to ultimate failure. Not carrying the one, multiplying instead of dividing, or factoring numerals in the wrong order seem like simple errors, but they all lead the student down a different pathway and to the incorrect solution.

The same can be said about Parkinson's patients and their personal pathways. Without a proper formula or plan of action, a Parkinson's patient can find themselves spinning their wheels in frustration while searching for a shred of consistency in their daily life. Something as simple as taking a pill only an hour later than scheduled, not getting in the daily walk in the neighborhood or on the treadmill, or not reaching a step goal for a given day can throw everything out of kilter and cause an unsuccessful day. However, instead of only having to grab an eraser and rework the problem on the paper, a simple error in the daily routine of a Parkinson's patient can potentially have more dire consequences. Minor missteps along the Parkinson's pathway can lead to longer off periods featuring more uncontrolled tremors, a sluggish feeling leading to the mental discomfort and frustration of not meeting a set daily routine, or in the worst case, physical or biological reactions to medicine (or lack thereof) in the system. The good news is, all this can be averted with the presence of a strong personal formula.

*****

Hannibal Smith from the classic TV series *The A-Team* was known for his famous catchphrase "I love it when a plan comes together." Parkinson's patients would be in full agreement with Hannibal but probably would not want to be involved with all the gadgets and physical fortitude he needed to survive some of the less conventional plans he concocted on the show. Instead, just having a solid formula or plan in place for surviving the daily rigors of the Parkinson's pathway is often comforting enough to get by. Personally, this second pillar of my Parkinson's journey is usually not as challenging for me to maintain, but I do recognize the potential pitfalls it brings for others. Even I struggle with the occasional difficulties this pillar presents from time to time.

What makes this particular aspect of Parkinson's life challenging is that while it is easy for some to create a plan, carrying it out and staying persistent with it until the end is often a formidable task. I compare it to making New Year's resolutions. In late December, when the finances are stretched by Christmas credit card bills and your waistline is stretched by all the goodies surrounding you on an hourly basis, it's quite easy to tell yourself, "I'm going to do better and save more money next year" or "I'm going to get over all this and lose weight next year." Simple. You've declared your mission, and you are eager to get underway. But we all know what happens to most of us. By the end of January, we are back at the department stores or loading up our carts on Amazon with "necessities," or we find ourselves justifying "just one more" doughnut for breakfast (to accompany the other three you've already consumed). By February, we are still in debt and still out of shape and wondering what happened to our formula for success. It then becomes easy to give up (or maybe that should read "give in") and throw our hands in the air, declaring we will "do better next year." Of course, we all know what will happen!

Why does this happen to some people while others seem to have no issues with successfully creating and meeting their goals in life? What does this tell us as Parkinson's patients? I think the connection between the two is clear. It is easy to make a *goal*, but it is more challenging to create a *plan* that will allow you to achieve that goal. In regard to the resolutions example, it is far easier to say "I want to save more money next year" than it is to sit down, analyze your family budget, and create specific, measurable steps that will lead you to that goal of saving money. The ones with strong formulas in place will not only generally declare their intentions to save more money; they will write down specific statements such as "I will eat out two fewer days each week this month" or "I will set up an automatic transaction with my bank to move 5 percent of my paycheck to a savings account each month." With specific steps outlined, it is much easier to track your progress toward a goal. Doing so keeps your focus on the steps along the journey instead of the finish line in the distance. I also compare it to running a 5K race. It is much simpler for me to tell myself during a race "Just make it to the next corner" or "You can make it for two more minutes" instead of thinking about the remaining two miles to go before finishing. Keeping my focus on the immediate surroundings and the incremental steps along the way keeps me on track to finish and allows me to enjoy the small successes along the way that are needed to get me to the finish line.

For a Parkinson's patient, the applications are similar. All patients know there will be struggles and complications along the pathway. That is a given. It's easy for me to declare "I just want to feel better this week" and then wonder why it doesn't magically happen that way. Many days I wake up thinking this will be the day things turn around for me. The tremors will be fewer and farther between. The side effects of my medicine will not be an issue. I'll be more rested and have more energy. It will be a great day! However, that mentality is flawed if it stands on its own. It is not enough for me to tell myself as many generalities as I can in order to have a good day. Achieving that goal requires a plan of specific and measurable steps. Instead of wishing for fewer tremors, I can work toward achieving that goal by making sure to take the proper meds at the proper intervals and set a goal of a certain number of steps each hour that can be tracked on my Apple Watch. Instead of hoping for no side effects from my pills, I can write out a daily menu for myself to make sure I have the correct balance of nutrition that will help counteract any nausea for the day. Instead of wishing for more energy, I create and adhere to a bedtime routine of getting to bed by 9:00 p.m. on school nights and 10:00 p.m. on weekends in order to get the required amount of rest so that I can operate more efficiently during the day. In more cliché language, failing to plan is the same thing as planning to fail.

For this second pillar, I have categorized my discoveries into three categories: medicine, motion, and mental health. Hopefully, sharing some experiences and portions of my plan for daily Parkinson's life will enable others to create formulas of their own in order to help make their journey a bit more manageable. Remember, each person has their own pathway through this experience, so a personal plan needs to be developed that best fits your own situation. One of the frustrating components of this disease is its variability. What impacts one patient at a certain stage might not impact another. The side effects one patient encounters might not be of the same severity as someone else's. The important thing is to find a formula that works for you and helps you make it through the daily journey.

Medicine. One of the more challenging aspects of my journey through Parkinson's has been with my medications. I am not one of those people who handle nausea or other stomach distress situations well at all, so if that is listed as a side effect on any pills I might have to take, it worries me. To put it mildly, I am not a good patient or a pleasant person to be around in a nauseated condition. I know plenty of people who, when they are ill, don't even mind throwing up. In fact, I think they look forward to it. Not me! I don't care how much better it might make me feel; I do not want to stick my head in the toilet and retch out my guts even once if I can avoid it.

That being the case, I needed a solid plan of action for taking my Parkinson's medicine that every label I read included the words "May cause nausea in some people" on it. Perhaps the biggest obstacle for me to overcome in this stage was the mental battle. My wife constantly reminded me to simply take the pill and not work myself up so much about it that I make myself sick. If I could convince myself that I wasn't going to have nausea, that might be half the battle. That, of course, was easier said than done.

The struggles with my lower dosages of carbidopa and levodopa in the initial months of my treatment had me concerned when they first hit. However, I soon managed to accept the dosages better when I would distract myself with something else at the prescribed time of my medication. That distraction could be watching something on TV or having a conversation with my wife or daughters, anything to keep my mind off what I was taking. At work, it was easier to get distracted. Being surrounded by energetic teenagers all day naturally keeps your mind off what you are doing in the moment. As long as I did not have the opportunity to think about getting sick, I was in decent shape. It did not always work, but it was a good formula to have in place.

As I have advanced through my journey a bit further in recent months, a new version of the challenge with nausea emerged. This one showed itself as I was going through battles with the gagging attacks. If I had an aversion to feeling nauseated before this time, it was surely made even worse in this portion of my existence. After I had battled these dry-heave-style attacks for several weeks, Dr. Raju altered my meds to my current dosage of carbidopa and levodopa (which is triple the dosage I started with after the initial diagnosis). He also gave me a nausea pill that has worked wonders.

After visiting my GI doctor and having my throat stretched, my condition improved dramatically to its current status where I only take one or two of the nausea pills each month. This beats the one or two I was taking each day just to get through work without puking in my classroom or in the office. Those were unpleasant times! I credit most of my success in this area to having a strict formula in place that allows me to schedule and arrange what I am going to eat and when to do so in order to correlate with the times to take my medications. It gets a bit crazy some days as my school lunch schedule is not a fixed point in time. But with a little planning (and the help of a mini fridge in the office), I make sure to have the right snacks and food available to get me through the workday with minimal issues. Even my students have commented to me that they have seen a change in my demeanor in class lately. I bet! There's no telling how rough I looked on those days when I had no sleep or was fighting nausea on a constant basis. It was all about the formula.

Motion. If the medicine was a challenging area for me in my adjustment to being diagnosed with Parkinson's, creating a formula or plan to remain in motion was just the opposite. From the first few days and weeks after my diagnosis up until the last few months, finding ways to stay in motion was easy. I would go on walks through the neighborhood almost every day, or I would go to the gym and get on the treadmill or the stationary bike and get my work in. Even when it seemed easy to do, it still required a formula that met certain criteria. In the fall semester, these days were easy to locate as my after-school responsibilities were minimal. All I had to do was figure out which days I actually wanted to exercise, put those dates into my phone, and then get it done. I live off my phone calendar, so having my exercise times already there was a no-brainer. Still, in creating these calendars, I had to be smart and reasonable. I could not schedule nine days in a row in the gym. I was dedicated, but not crazy! Often, I would schedule a gym treadmill session when a ball game was on so that I could watch it while exercising. That made it seem as if the time was going by faster.

During my running streak of 5K races, the formula was even easier. I would schedule and pay for races five or six weeks in advance and put them in my phone. There was no way I was going to miss those. The longer the streak lasted, the more determined I was to keep it going. There were a couple of weekends where I had to scramble to find a Sunday afternoon 5K in some remote location an hour or so from home just to keep the streak alive. I even found a race that only had twenty-five people in it, and the registration prize was a cat food dish. That made more sense after I realized it was a fundraising event for a local humane society shelter. No matter the type of event, I knew that with proper planning and some logistical arrangements, the streak would continue and my formula to keep myself moving would be intact.

As easy as this formula was to create and follow in the early and middle stages of my Parkinson's journey, it has become more challenging in the last few months. Once the streak was broken, the push to run in order to keep the streak alive was gone. I had to find other motivation, and that was (and still is) not easy for me. The streak ended in late summer of 2020, and I justified that nobody in their right mind wants to run in August and September in Georgia. Why would someone do that? Of course, I was forgetting that I had done just that a year ago with no real concerns. As it stands for me at this point in time, I am looking at some local 5K races to get back in the groove again. I keep having to remind myself that anyone can create a goal, but not just anyone can envision and formulize the needed incremental steps to get to that goal. As I continue with this struggle, maybe I need to go back to following my own advice. Don't focus on the 3.1 miles between you and the finish line, take the journey one small step at a time, and enjoy the small successes along the way.

Along with running and walking, I have found golf to be a wonderful part of my formula to stay in motion. I can thank Coach Gary Richey for this one as he helped me line up a spot with him coaching the golf teams at school. I would be the middle school head coach and an assistant coach for the varsity. This allowed me to go out on the course with the guys and gals on all the teams, spend time on the driving range with them, play nine holes about three times a week, and then walk some really challenging courses with them when they played in weekend tournaments. It wasn't long before I was noticing an improved sense of mobility off the course as well. I created a plan to video my swings at least once a week on the range. I found that within about two to three weeks, I was getting more range of motion on my backswing and my grip was getting stronger. This works out well for my work schedule as it gets my golf game into some kind of form before the summer break starts, and more time opens up on my calendar to play. I used to kid around and tell people my doctor actually prescribed more golf as part of my treatment. Looking back at how this portion of the formula for motion has worked out, maybe it wasn't as big a joke as I originally thought.

Mental state. Creating a formula to improve your mental state may seem easy at first, but the challenges reveal themselves as you dig down into the dirty details of trying to put this into practice. Most people would agree that mental health issues are a growing concern in our nation and across the world as well. With the isolation and frustrations brought on by the COVID-19 pandemic, people do not get the societal exposure needed to maintain good mental health. In my case, I was already an introvert, so the pandemic did more to validate my behavior than show me a drastic need to change it. I could teach remotely from my home office, be done as soon as the final bell sounded, and never have to physically cross paths with another human being throughout the entire workday. At times, I felt great about this setup. After a while, though, the stark reality of the situation began to set in. While I often used my Parkinson's condition as a crutch and an excuse to maintain my "glorified hermit" status in the world, I was slowly beginning to realize that I had to do more. I had to discover a way to break out of my virtual shell and reengage the outside world, even if it meant being masked in order to do it.

I found my formula for maintaining my mental state by accepting three realities as truth in my world. First, I might have Parkinson's, but it is not going to kill me. Second, I am the only one in complete control of my emotional state. Third, I do not need to be afraid to say "I don't know" when confronted with a new challenge or question that rattles me. Keeping these three realities in the forefront allows me to take charge of my own mental progress instead of letting someone or something else hijack and throw me off course so badly that I leave my pathway and cannot find my way back.

First, I have Parkinson's, but it is not going to kill me. For a short while after my initial diagnosis, I viewed it as a death sentence. I was going to shrivel up to nothing, crawl into my bed, hide from the outside world, and wait for the end to come. It took me some time to work through that stage, but it was Dr. Raju who reminded me that there were many other medical conditions with which I could have been diagnosed that would be much worse. It could have been an inoperable cancer. I could have had a massive heart attack, and that would have been it right then and there. The doctor always made it a point to remind me that what I had was not curable, but it was treatable to the point where my quality of life could be maintained at a decent level. I just needed to accept the fact that life was going to be challenging, but it would not be impossible. Sooner or later, I would have to realize I had it better than many people around me.

Second, I am the only one in control of my mental state. This is a tough one to accept because of the enormous amounts of external factors constantly working on us in our daily lives. It would be easy to see the "beautiful people" in the ads or on TV shows and wonder why I can't have their life. I want the big house with the huge yard, the endless bank accounts, and the love and admiration of all the people around me. Sadly, this is not my reality. Life for me is more like a collection of flat tires, broken air filters, screaming children, and the dream that one of these days my family and I will get to take a real vacation…somewhere…anywhere! Once I accepted the fact that my life had changed due to Parkinson's but it had not ended, I was in a much better place to move forward. If I wanted to be in a good mood, it was up to me to make that happen. In a way, it is my choice to enjoy the walk down my pathway. I can either focus on the potential doom and gloom that might be on all sides of my pathway, be jealous of the fabulous yet fake lives of the "beautiful people," or I can tell myself each day that I am simply going to try to make this one better than the last one. If I focus on my own responsibilities in this process, I can more quickly accept control of my own mood and, thus, my own metal condition.

Third, I do not need to be afraid to say "I don't know." It's a natural reaction for me to fear the unknown. As a Parkinson's patient, I often feel overwhelmed with things for which I have no answer. What will my tremors be like in class this week when I need to deliver an important lecture and review to my students? Will I be able to control my shaking? Will they notice? Will they care? Wondering about such things does me no good. I know this, but I still do it anyway because it's easy! There are days when I try to envision my future self at age sixty or seventy. If I stay on my current levels of progression, how difficult will life be? Will I even still be here? The answer to all these distracting concerns is, "I don't know." Those can be hard words to say to yourself or out loud because it means that we might not have everything together, as if that were a requirement in today's society. Instead of worrying about some scenario over which I have no control and that is going to happen whether I like it or not, I choose to focus more of my energy on the present. Doing this increases the likelihood that my formulas will be more fully developed and that I will be successful in the immediate time frames of my journey. In turn, these more immediate smaller successes lead to larger ones and, in turn, can help reduce the number of items that fall into the category of the unknown.

Three immediate realities lie between you and control of your own mental state as a Parkinson's patient. In no way do I claim to have mastered or entirely integrated these concepts into my life. It is a daily struggle but one that I know I can survive as long as I keep my wits about me and make sure the formula is in place. Going back to the example of my younger brother's hieroglyphic-style math problems, I don't have to understand everything about them and their construction. I can appreciate the solution and work on digesting the integral parts at a pace that is most manageable for me. I may never fully understand the concepts and the logic behind the problem, but I can rest assured there is a solution, and I am making daily progress toward discovering it more fully.

Pillar Number 3—Flexibility

It's pretty safe to say I do not like change. If you give me a schedule, a roster, an agenda, or a to-do list with a deadline, I am happy. I am the type of person who goes to the grocery store with a list, knows right where to go to find the items on the shelves, gathers the items, stacks them neatly in the cart (yes, there is a science and a "proper" way to put your items into the cart), and then heads to the checkout where like items are grouped together as much as possible. After completing the transaction, the bags need to be carefully placed back in the cart and then hauled to the car. Once there, the back seat is the only option for storage of the said items. Putting them in the trunk means risking them shifting uncontrollably and potentially spilling out and rolling all around. It's a sickness, I guess, but one that I proudly lay claim to. No, I really do not like change!

My daughters call it man shopping. It's even worse, they tell me, when I have to go to the mall. I want to park close to the store, go right in, get what I need, pay, and get out. They, on the other hand, seem to have no natural compass embedded in their brains as they enjoy wandering aimlessly and browsing in no real sequence. They will occasionally decide to visit a store at the completely other end of the mall even though we just passed by that store a few minutes ago. Frustrating! One should have a routine and stick to it. Don't interrupt my favorite show for a "special report" at the most critical point in the plot. Yes, I'm sure the tragic plane crash in Asia that's being reported on is awful, but I need to know how the show is going to turn out!

The same semblance of order applies to my journey through Parkinson's. While it might have taken me longer than it should to finally discover the routine that best suits my condition, now that the routine is there, I do everything I can to adhere to it. Pills every five hours? Check! Eating food with my medication? Check! Record and track my sleep with an iPhone app? Check! At times, my entire life seems like one big checklist. Get up at 5:00 a.m. Leave for work by 5:45 a.m. Teach from 8:30 a.m. until 4:00 p.m. Get home by 5:00 p.m. Dinner by 6:00 p.m. In bed at 9:00 p.m. Repeat again tomorrow. It's a simple and, at times, boring existence, but it's all mine, and I like things to go a certain way. Please do not ask me to do something not previously scheduled unless it's an emergency or something with which I can create a suitable work-around so that my schedule gets realigned to its proper balance as soon as possible.

This type of life is probably what drew me into my introverted existence and aided my bouts with depression before I discovered the issue and took steps to correct it. I could schedule myself into doing nothing. That might sound impossible, but I could content myself with just bumming out on the couch, watching games involving teams I might not even care about if it meant I could explain this to my family as needing some downtime. I'm sure my wife and kids probably thought if I had any more downtime, I'd never get up again! They were probably not wrong on many occasions.

Working my way through my Parkinson's pathway, I have discovered the need for flexibility in two areas: mental and physical. Each of these two areas holds their own challenges and requirements, but for me to be at my best and to continue to make progress in my journey, I have found that I must be able to adjust myself in those two key areas in order to not only be a better and more successful Parkinson's patient but to also be a better husband, father, colleague, friend, and overall person. Having success in only one of these two areas is not enough to be able to consider myself successful. I might, at times, find one of the two areas more convenient or manageable, but it cannot be done at the expense of the other.

For example, there are days when I know I will be more physically active. It could be a 5K race, a round of golf, or just a challenging and hectic day at school with a thousand errands to run and student conferences to conduct. On those days, I realize going in the need to be physically more flexible and mobile with my body. In order to accomplish that goal, I must do all the little things right: take the correct pills, eat the right meals, stretch and keep moving at the right times. It's not usually difficult to manage those responsibilities, and it becomes even easier when I tell myself that I will actually feel better during and after these physical exertions if I do those little things correctly. But even experiencing a high level of success with my physical flexibility does not make the entire Parkinson's experience a success if my emotional or mental experiences are not equally successful. I could play eighteen holes of golf and have a high degree of range of motion, but if I am not attuned to enjoying the experience and remaining positive with my team members and colleagues, then the progress made in my physical flexibility is for naught.

One of the key moments in my journey was a day in March of 2020 about two weeks before our school shut down face-to-face learning and went all virtual. On that day, I had a new experience while teaching my classes. I found it almost impossible to "talk with my hands" and reach and point toward my classroom video screen. The physical movement of my hands and arms just wasn't happening. I normally move my hands a great deal while I am teaching. On that day, though, I resorted to teaching with my arms folded or with my hands in my pockets. I'm sure it looked strange to my kids in class, but it was better to teach in what might have been the only posture that seemed comfortable at the time than to continually stretch out an unstable hand or arm to the screen and feel even more self-conscious about that. It was a frustrating experience that led directly to my reengagement with Dr. Raju and the new prescriptions of medications that have since led to a much more comfortable teaching experience for me. There are still days when I will teach from my desk, perched in my chair, but I would like to believe that is more of a result of me trying to remain socially distanced from my students than trying to compensate for a lack of physical flexibility or mobility.

Another key moment in which my lack of flexibility created a bit of a panic on my part was in the fall semester of 2019. Up until that time, I had always told myself that I was lucky to have not experienced major difficulty in my morning routine of getting ready and getting dressed because of my Parkinson's condition. Things started to change that semester as I would find myself unable to button my shirt without a major ordeal that created frustration and anger more often than it did a properly buttoned shirt. The same was holding true with the fasteners on my slacks. My wife came to the rescue on both accounts as she knew how unraveled I would get just trying to do something simple like getting dressed in the morning. In a matter of a couple of days, Becky added Velcro fasteners to my shirts so that they would press closed and still look like they had been buttoned properly. She also added sliding clasps to my pants for work, so there was no longer any need to button them. Such simple fixes but enormous rewards. Yes, the medications were helping with my dexterity also, but not having to get all worked up about getting dressed for school in the mornings was the best medicine of all. I have my loving wife and her ingenuity to thank for that! Her actions aided me in my physical flexibility but, maybe more importantly, aided me in the second category as well—my mental flexibility.

It is a given that Parkinson's patients are going to have to deal with limited physical flexibility and find ways to deal with that issue, but we also have to face the fact that we are going to suffer through a lack of mental flexibility as well. This can reveal itself in a couple of ways. First, and perhaps most obviously, limited mental flexibility can show up in neurological symptoms, such as struggling with memory loss and mild forms of dementia. Additionally, I have read that almost half of all Parkinson's sufferers experience some form of hallucinations from time to time. While these issues are related to and attack the brain and neural components of Parkinson's patients, I don't necessarily see them as the predominant issue involving mental flexibility. I feel this way because they can be made more tolerable through medical or psychological treatments. In some ways, then, these mental flexibility limitations are also rooted in the physical condition.

Perhaps mental flexibility involves more than just making chemical neurological adjustments. For me, it involves keeping myself open to others and their environments instead of shining life's spotlight only on me and my limitations. Just because I have Parkinson's does not mean that I have to sentence myself to a deathbed, dreary lifestyle. I can choose to meet the challenge head-on and find ways to be flexible with my time and my attitude in order to be more helpful to others. As soon as I close the door on the outside world, not only do I limit what interaction others can have with me that could prove beneficial for me but I also limit the degree of interaction I can have with others in an attempt to help them in some way.

I'll admit…this is a really tough one for me to get right. Even before my Parkinson's diagnosis, I know I was more centered on myself than I should have been. If I did not want to do something, I did not do it. I was the world's best at saying no to things. I was just as happy staying within my own little world, and I did not see the need to expand my horizons too far in any direction. In some ways, my diagnosis gave me an additional crutch or excuse to continue acting that way. I would convince myself I couldn't do something because I had Parkinson's, and it might be difficult. I was afraid to try. I was afraid to take a leap of faith. I'm not even sure that's right. It wasn't just a leap of faith that scared me; it was making a single hop, skip, or jump in any direction that caused me to want to do my best roly-poly impersonation and curl up in a little ball in the corner and hope nobody wanted to step on me and squash my world.

For me, my most challenging experience in mental flexibility is the moment when my alarm clock goes off at 5:00 a.m. on a school day and it's time to get the process started for another day of teaching teenagers. In my better moments, I roll right out of the bed and know exactly how the morning is going to go. There's no groaning, no mental debate, no lingering toe or leg cramps from the night before. It's just a normal start to a normal day, and it's time to get moving. My worst mental flexibility moments are spotted a mile away. They usually begin with me telling myself how awful I slept that night or tracking how many different hours on the clock I had seen since going to bed. Of course, this self-discussion was taking place without me having moved a muscle in the direction of getting upright on the floor and heading for the bathroom. The debate was on in full force. Do I go into work or not? What am I really experiencing? What would happen if I didn't go in? Do I have a lesson or video in place for the kids? Once again, this is all taking place with me *still* in a prone position and staring at the clock now reading 5:01…5:02…5:05!

These moments are not at all like the mornings after nights in which I suffered physical issues such as tremors, gagging attacks, or other issues that had me wiped out and often still in some degree of pain. Those days were easier to manage because there was no need for mental gymnastics involving working or not working that day. If I couldn't function, I couldn't function, and that was that. These days were different. I had to convince myself that I could do this thing called life and get through it no matter what. Many mornings, I won the debate and got things rolling as close to the usual pattern as possible. Some mornings, though, I was not up to the mental wrestling match with myself and gave in to the mental distress signals and called it a day. I'm not proud of those moments, but I have become much better at winning those mental flexibility battles with the help of the new medications in my prescriptions. The increased confidence and, dare I say, energy from the new regimen have given me a leg up on my own mental flexibility and have allowed me more victorious moments in the past six months than I had in the previous three years combined. The famous New York Yankees catcher Yogi Berra once said, "Ninety percent of this game is half mental." As unusual as that proverb is, there is some truth to it for a Parkinson's patient. There's medicine for the physical ailments and symptoms of Parkinson's. There may even be medicines to help patients get a bit better grasp of their chemical and neurological balances. But one thing remains true. Only the Parkinson's patient themselves can fight to win the battle of mental flexibility.

The next time you go into a grocery store, think about your experience. Do you have the physical flexibility to manually maneuver your way through the aisles and reach items on the top shelf? Are you constrained in any way? If not, say a prayer of thankfulness.

However, also ask yourself if you can conquer the mental experience I experience in the store. Do you have to arrange items in your cart just so? Do you always follow your list? Do you group like items at the checkout? If so, your mental flexibility, like mine, may need some work! I tell you what. I'll continue to work on gaining confidence in helping others and adjusting the use of my time. I think I'm more likely to have success in that area of my flexibility than I am about arranging the bag of marshmallows a safe distance from the heavy carton of sodas in the basket or placing all the canned items safely in the bottom-right corner of the cart. Everyone's got to have something to work on, I guess!

Pillar Number 4—Finish!

In 2012, I set a goal for myself to run a marathon. At the time, it sounded like a good idea. I thought to myself, *It's only 26.2 miles. It can't be that bad! Thousands of people do this every year. Surely I can be one of them.* In July of that year, I bought the best marathon training book I could find and read it cover to cover in just a few days. It had training logs, nutritional plans, tips on what shoes to get, and just about everything else you might need to make it to the finish line. I had my plan; now all I needed was to find the right racecourse. My internet searches led me to three possibilities: the New York City Marathon, the Chicago Marathon, or the Disney Marathon in Orlando. All were great courses. All had tradition. But one of them had items of particular interest to my twelve-year-old twin girls—Mickey Mouse and princesses! So the Disney Marathon in January of 2013 would be it. Family vacation and my first marathon all in one package.

Training started immediately. Of course, marathon training in Georgia in July is not a wise option most days. I discovered how much I hate humidity. Training runs were done in the predawn hours or late at night for the summer months. As the runs got longer throughout the training, I would tell myself "Just one more mile" or "One more lap" around my training course. That motivation worked most days, but there were those off days when my mantra changed to "Just get to the next stop sign" or "Can you get to the end of the block?" Those were difficult days, but I learned the value of breaking more daunting larger tasks down into manageable segments that allowed me to enjoy success along the way. Soon, the months of training were done. On my last training run, I remembered one of the tips from the book—don't ever run the full 26.2 miles on a training run if you're attempting your first marathon. The author was convinced that the euphoria of completing that distance should be reserved for the real finish line of the race. So my last run was 26.1 miles, and I was ready to go.

It was a 5:00 a.m. start time, so I was up at 2:00 a.m. and headed to the start line. Nerves were jumping, but it was energetic in a way. Thousands of people were lined up in their corrals, waiting for the gun to sound. It did, and away we all went, running through all the Disney parks on our way to the finish line at Epcot. I remembered my training and settled in at a nice, even pace. Five miles done! Ten miles done! Then 13.1 miles done! Halfway there and only a mild sense of discomfort a couple of times that was remedied by eating my energy gel gummies. I was growing in confidence as I turned the corner into the Wide World of Sports Complex, and then it happened—leg cramps that would have brought down an elephant! It was right at the mile marker 20, and I was in trouble! I walked about half a mile and worked out the pain, aided by my electrolytes in the drinks I was carrying. I was about to get going again when a gentleman about my age slowed down beside me to check on me. I told him I was good to go. He did not seem convinced and asked if he could tag along with me. Sounded good to me. For the next two miles, we jogged at a leisurely pace and talked about the course and the training we had done. Before I knew it, my leg strength was back to normal and I could get back closer to my normal pace. I asked my new running buddy if he wanted to go ahead. He said no but told me to "get after it" and "finish strong." Just about three miles later, I was in Epcot and closing in on the finish line, and soon this would all be done. In a truly non-world-record time of 5:15:26, I crossed the finish line and met my goal. It was easily the most amazing feeling I had ever experienced, and I owed a good portion of gratitude to my "guardian angel" at mile 20.

*****

In much the same way as training for and enduring my first marathon, my Parkinson's journey has offered many challenges, obstacles, and encouraging moments. From that initial day of diagnosis and all the confusion, fear, and uncertainty it brought to the overwhelming support and kindness from family, friends, and colleagues, living with Parkinson's has enabled me to experience a wide range of emotions.

Like the nervous energy of the marathon starting line, I have days and moments when I am excited about progress I am making physically or when the medications are working the way they are supposed to. There's always a bit of hesitation when things are going well. In the same way that my strength and confidence was building in the opening miles of the marathon, my confidence and strength grows on the "good days" I experience on my Parkinson's pathway. Of course, there are other times where the experience is not so encouraging.

As in the marathon when muscles began to ache and cramps were trying their hardest to make me give in, my Parkinson's journey has had its fair share of rough times as well. Sleepless nights, rampant battles with nausea, tremors that never seem to want to subside, and the depressive moments when I just wanted to curl up under the covers and not face the healthy people of the world on that particular day were my obstacles. They would slow me down, make me question any previous progress I had made, and bring me to a near standstill in certain moments. However, they have not forced me to quit the race or give up.

In times when I need a Parkinson's "running buddy," someone is always there. It might be my wife, who knows just what to say or, as is needed sometimes, when to kick me in the seat of my pants and get me going again. It could be a text or Facebook post from someone with an encouraging word or them taking a moment just to check in on me in that moment. These "running buddies" or, better named, "guardian angels" are the real reason I can continue in the race down the pathway. If only we were all as lucky as I am to have those people who tell me to "get after it" and "finish strong."

This fourth and final pillar of my Parkinson's pathway is centered around three encouragements I try to keep in mind along my journey. These statements have helped me in difficult times for sure, but they are better used as tools to keep me focused on the pathway instead of becoming distracted by all the potential surrounding distractions. During a race, it is easy to get sidetracked as people pass by you, your shoelace comes undone, the course winds its way up a steep hill that seems to go on forever, or you are just plain tired. I find that by keeping these encouraging words in mind, my "race" becomes more about the moment instead of me or the finish line. If I learn to enjoy and take advantage of the moment, the journey will be a success. A marathon has a set finish line. It's a glorious sight for a runner after pounding the pavement for hours. It gives a burst of renewed energy to the competitor and beckons them to complete their journey. While my Parkinson's pathway does not have a true finish line in that sense because there is currently no cure for it, I find that establishing multiple finish lines along the way works well. If crossing a finish line in a marathon equals success, then imagine if you could experience multiple successes in one journey. No, you don't have to run multiple marathons in order to get that experience. Instead, you establish the short-term goals as finish lines and cross them as many times as possible. I'll never win a marathon, but I can call myself a winner on the pathway of my Parkinson's experience if I find my own successes and help others along the way to do the same.

Statement 1: Stay the course. During my training, everything did not always go as planned. Some days I skipped out on runs when I just couldn't drag myself out of the house to get the work in. Other times, I would be on a training run and feel pretty good for the first mile or so, but then shin splints, leg cramps, or some other issue showed up, and I would end up cutting my run short. Sometimes I even turned right around where I was and walked back to the house. While there were bad days and disappointing moments during the training, I would always find my way to get back on track. I'd lace up the shoes once again and get back on the roads and find my way through my training. It was not always a pretty sight or an efficient run, but I stayed on the course and got the work in so I would be ready for the big day in Orlando. If I had not stayed the course and had allowed myself to give up, there's no way I would have been able to manage the 26.2 racecourse in Disney. Lesson learned: put in the work, dedicate the time, follow the course markings, and finish the race!

The same principle applies to my journey through Parkinson's. I can't tell you how many days I have had where I just wanted to quit. I have wanted to be done with all the medical visits, prescription plans, life adjustments, and inconveniences of having Parkinson's. In all these times, I longed for the pre-Parkinson's days when mobility was not a central focus of my life and when I didn't carry around a small pharmacy with me pretty much everywhere I go. I remember days when I did not have to set alarms on my watch or phone to remind me to take a pill. I think about when sleep was just something that came naturally at the end of the day and not something that had to be tracked and monitored all the time. Yes, I have wanted to go back to those days on numerous occasions, but I can't.

Part of my learning to stay the course with Parkinson's is the ability to accept my current reality. It is true there is no cure for this disease, but I cannot live my life thinking that will always be true. I have to continue to be optimistic that a breakthrough might be coming in the near future that will alter my journey in some dramatic fashion. Even though I remain hopeful to see that day, I can't afford to dwell upon it. My pathway is always right in front of me, and I can't simply press pause and wait for better times or new breakthroughs in medicine. I have to figure out what lies immediately ahead of me and figure out how to deal with that first. I will admit I am not always as successful at this as I would like to be. I struggle at times putting one foot in front of the other and making it through the day. However, I know that I do not really have a choice. Life requires me to "lace up my sneakers" each day, step out into the reality of my pathway, scan the horizon for obstacles, and just keep moving. For me, staying the course means figuring out my routine, setting up a plan of attack, conquering the hills along the way, and following the "signs" laid out for me to make it toward the finish line. That finish line might just be the end of the next class period or the drive into work on a stressful traffic day, or it might be making it through a week of taking all my pills at the proper time. Whatever it looks like, I know my chances of reaching the established finish line are better if I continue to stay the course!

Statement 2: Pick yourself up. I've physically fallen only twice during a race. Both times, there was no one to blame but myself. The first time was in the Atlanta Track Club 10 Miler when I was not paying attention to my steps and the course conditions and stepped right in the middle of a pothole and went crashing down to the pavement. It was more embarrassing than painful, but it was a setback. The second time was during a race on the Suwanee Greenway. This flat, normally benign course got me when, once again, I was not thinking about being careful and slipped and fell on a slick spot on the path where water had gathered after a recent rain. I wish the stories were more dramatic, but those types of stories don't just happen to someone who is being careless or clumsy during a run. Instead, I just have to regain my composure and my stride, laugh it off, hope nobody was there recording the event on their cell phone, and then get back to the business at hand.

As a Parkinson's patient, I can relate to these stories of falling down and then having to keep going. Since I am an early onset Parkinson's patient and still in my first five years of living with the disease, physical falls are not really a challenge for me at this point. This is a blessing. I know, though, that the increased likelihood of balance issues and falls exists somewhere down the road of my journey as I have talked to those with Parkinson's who are experiencing those issues currently. To be honest, the falling is one of things that scares me the most about my future in Parkinson's. Losing control of my balance and being unsteady does not seem like a desirable condition. Being in that state would definitely limit my running and could also impact my terrible golf game to the point of maybe keeping me off the course. While that might be safer for the other golfers on the course when I am playing, it would be frustrating for me to experience.

Just because I am not physically falling at this stage of Parkinson's does not mean I have no need to "pick myself up" from "down" times. I might not have toppled down a set of stairs or lost my balance in the classroom and missed my chair behind my desk, but I have "fallen" just as much as any wobbling toddler, but in my own way. On days when the tremors are at their worst and the medications are not kicking in as swiftly or effectively as I would like, I will get so frustrated with the experience that I will (sometimes violently) grab my left arm or left leg and pin it down. This pinning is usually accompanied by significant grumbling and the occasional choice word or two. If I don't pin them down, I'll get off my chair and pace the floor to work out the twitching and instability. Of course, this also has to be partnered with the appropriate amount of mumbling and complaining (sometimes to no one in particular) for it to be a complete experience.

No matter the circumstances, I am always faced with the same choice. I can either stay in a collapsed state and bemoan my unfortunate circumstances, or I can just get through it and move on to the next segment of the journey. Falling on the racecourse and then just lying there and doing nothing will not get me where I want to go. It might be more comfortable and, in some weird way, more satisfying to stay where I am, watching the others go hurtling by while I throw my own little pity party on the side of the course. I know, though, that is not the option I can choose. If I need a moment to regroup and assess the situation, that's fine. What I can't do is refuse to get back up and keep moving. There is a race to finish, goals to be met, and successes to be experienced. If I stay on the sidelines, I might not get to experience some unexpected success like running a personal best in the next mile or finishing higher up in my age-group than before. Sure, it's easy to stay down, but it takes a competitor to get back up.

In my Parkinson's experience, I have stayed down before and not enjoyed the result. All the times I was so frustrated with my medicines making me sick or not working the way I thought they should served to knock me down consistently. I finally began refusing to fight back. It was the equivalent of taking off my sneakers during a race and giving up. These experiences in my Parkinson's journey led me closer to the depressed state I found myself in during 2018 and 2019. I was down and depressed, but I did not really grasp the severity of my situation. In a way, I was enjoying being down on the side of the pathway, watching others run by in their effortless strides, while all I wanted to do was take off my race number, turn off the headphones, and just go back home. It took my wife and family holding a mirror up to my life for me to see what was truly going on and how long I had been "on the side of the road." With their encouragement, I got the sneakers laced back up and got back in the race. I might not have reached the ultimate finish line yet, but I am up and moving again. I'll continue setting those incremental goals and enjoying small victories. I'm sure I will fall again, but it won't be the end of my race. I'll take a moment, reassess, and then pick myself up and keep going!

Statement 3: Help someone else along the way. Runners definitely feel part of a community. No matter what the race or skill level, everyone in the event seems to pull for everyone else. In smaller 5K races, I can usually tell which runners are going to be the ones to beat. Even those better runners still take time to cheer everyone else on after they have finished. It's a part of the sport I admire and enjoy the most. Trying to beat my own times or get a better qualifying spot for a future race is fun, but seeing well-established runners staying around and cheering those who are at the back of the pack as they come down the stretch is a wonderful sight. It's something I wish more people could take and apply to everyday life.

I have also been fortunate to meet some really nice people at the races I have done. About a year ago, I met Rusty at a local 5K race, and he and I have run numerous races together. Rusty is older than I am but still manages to beat me in just about every race we compete in together. He has his own "team" of "brunch bunch" runners that he has developed and introduced me to along the way. The people I have met through him are wonderful, down-to-earth folks who enjoy the running community. I have also met fellow Parkinson's patients in these races and have enjoyed hearing their stories and how they battle along their own personal pathways as I do.

This community aspect also applies to my Parkinson's journey. In the last five years, I have been blessed to be in a support group through a local church. The group consisted of five to six people who all have Parkinson's. I have to admit, going to the meetings in this group definitely made me feel young as I was the youngest one there by about twenty years or so. These gentlemen are very encouraging and have offered great insights into what is down the road apiece for me in my journey. Their wives would also meet at the same time as us and share support stories and discuss their roles in our lives. We surely would not be as well off as we are if we did not have amazing women standing behind us, caring for us, and supporting us through all the challenges we have faced.

Having seen the importance of these communities of support, I have come to realize something. It is wonderful to be the one on the receiving end of these supporters, but it is also an equally rewarding experience to be the one to find someone else who is suffering and help bring them along down the pathway. It may not be possible to lead them down the exact same pathway you are on, but you can surely help them see the guideposts on their own pathway and steer them in the right direction with an encouraging word or a message at just the right time and place. It is for this very reason that I have made it a point to stick around at least for a few minutes at each race when I can and encourage those finishing behind me. I know how much that means to me, and I want to be able to pass it along. That same reasoning is what led me to craft this section of my story. I might not know exactly what an individual's challenge is on their own Parkinson's pathway, but if sharing my story and insights from my experience can help one individual take a step in the right direction, then all this writing has been worth it. I will continue to seek out runners to cheer for at my races, but I also hope these stories and thoughts I have provided here will help someone else to be encouraged and, in turn, find another member of the Parkinson's community and reach out in order to support them. If we all work together, then we can all find the finish line of our own Parkinson's pathways!

ACKNOWLEDGMENTS

These are always dangerous pages to attempt because I know that I will probably leave somebody out who needs mentioning. Just know that those who have played a part in my story are all valued and appreciated more than you could ever know or that could be written on a single page. All of you have contributed to this work and have helped me in countless ways to make it through the first five years of my Parkinson's journey. I appreciate each and every one of you who have helped me reach this point, and I pray that your influence will continue to be felt in my life for many more years to come.

Having said that, there are people I would like to thank personally for their part in this project and for their support in my life. First and foremost, I would like to thank my loving wife, Becky, and my two amazing daughters, Summar and Savannah. There's no telling how much I have put you through in these five years, and I appreciate your undying love and support through all my grumbling, complaining, medical issues, and other things. You have all been right there for me when I needed you most, and I pray that I can continue to try to get better and be the best husband and father I can be for you three beautiful ladies.

I also want to thank my parents, Don and Elaine Hill, and my brothers, John and Stephen, for their support and prayers in this ordeal. Thank you for all the supportive phone calls, visits, Facebook comments, and "likes" of my photos throughout these five years. I appreciate your constant concern and support on my behalf. It is nice to know that I can always reach out if needed and find great support from my family, and I wish you all good health and good fortune in the years to come.

Finally, I would like to thank many of my colleagues from work at Greater Atlanta Christian School and my graduate school group from Piedmont College. At work, I would not have made it through without the incredible support and prayers from my officemates (past and present): Jami and Brad Denton, Jennifer Thomas, Lauri Fields, Tami Miller, Jeremy Beauchamp, Tammy Hughes, Ellie Kenworthy, Jenny Runkel, Savannah Roberts, Gary Richey, Bailey Baker, Delaney Craig, and Chris Sharp. This amazing team of colleagues has gone above and beyond the call of duty to be a prayer warrior group for me and for my family. They have covered classes, printed off materials, helped with subs, and did countless other tasks to help me in times of need. Thank you for all you have done and continue to do. I would be remiss if I did not also mention our amazing administrators who have helped me through some challenging times. Thanks to Shane Woodward (the best principal and friend a teacher could ask for), Robbie Wilson, Crystal Downs, Tina Martin, Joy Osgood, Charles Edwards, and the entire attendance staff who have helped arrange subs for me, sometimes at very late notice. You are all amazing parts of my journey, and I value your support and friendship.

From my Piedmont College group, I would like to thank Dr. David Sells and Dr. Nancy Kluge for your incredible help in getting me across that stage to get my doctorate. You are two of my most valued friends, and I appreciate all you have done for me and for my family. David, I also appreciate you missing all those putts in our friendly golf matches, allowing me to win! Thanks also to Dr. Charles Lucado, Dr. Karen Samuelsen, and Dr. McCullom for their encouragement and support in my doctoral adventures.

Hopefully, I haven't left out too many names. Rest assured that it takes a village to get someone like me down their Parkinson's pathway. I look forward to the continued support for many more years to come. I will not give up on this battle. I will continue this journey!

ABOUT THE AUTHOR

Dr. Gerry Hill has been a Parkinson's patient since 2016 when he was diagnosed with early onset Parkinson's disease at age forty-eight. A full-time educator, Dr. Hill continued teaching his high school English classes and finishing his doctorate while also fighting the daily struggles that come with Parkinson's. Dr. Hill has taught high school English for twenty-four years. He has been married to his wife, Becky, for the last thirty-one years and has twin daughters, Summar and Savannah, who are both in college. A native of Birmingham, Alabama, Dr. Hill has taught in Missouri as well as his current teaching position in Norcross, Georgia, at Greater Atlanta Christian School.

CPSIA information can be obtained
at www.ICGtesting.com
Printed in the USA
LVHW110330040821
694386LV00004B/198